Acupressure and Magnetotherapy

Acupressure and Magnetotherapy are two alternate systems of medicine which are drugless, noninvasive and have no side effects. They complement each other so well that they can be used together simultaneously for better results. These therapies are effective for both healing and preventing ailments. This self-help book is a guide to good health and wellness using these therapies.

These alternate systems require one to follow the laws of nature, irrespective of one's job profile, routine and working hours. The book provides both an introduction to acupressure and magnetotherapy as well as advice on: (a) proper breathing (b) balanced diet (c) proper sleep (d) regular elimination (f) adequate exercise (g) laughter for coping with stress. Since the body is a whole unit, the holistic approach is emphasized.

The therapies rely on knowledge gained from ancient scriptures. They rely heavily on balancing of the endocrine glands (also known as chakras in other systems). The prevention of ailments is primary. For this the use of magnets and magnetic healing water can hardly be over emphasized. Further, the regular pressing of master points, as prescribed in our therapy, helps ward off over 100 ailments. Pressing the points on the face enables one to know the state of the digestive system and has anti-ageing effects. Regular pressing of finger points also helps ward off many ailments. Most of these actions do not take more than a couple of minutes each. Not all need to be done together. Select a few and press them at your convenience. Healing is literally at your finger tips.

Acupressure and Magnetotherapy

Holistic Approach to Healing and Preventing Ailments

Wg.Cdr. (Retd.) Dr. Inder Puri VM & BAR

Dr. Chanda Seth

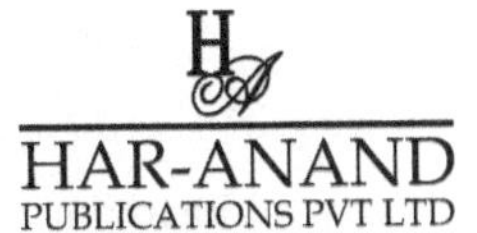

HAR-ANAND
PUBLICATIONS PVT LTD

Published by Ashok Gosain and Ashish Gosain for:
HAR-ANAND PUBLICATIONS PVT LTD
E-49/3, Okhla Industrial Area, Phase-II, New Delhi-110020
Tel.: 41603490
E-mail: info@haranandbooks.com/haranand@rediffmail.com
Shop online at: www.haranandbooks.com

Printed in India

Acknowledgements

This book is a distillation of my learnings from two decades of practice, research, workshops and experimentation in the field of Acupressure and Magnetotherapy as well as other alternative health systems. It has been my earnest endeavour to heal and prevent ailments related to the human body. My experience has enhanced my belief in the holistic approach to health.

In my practice I continue to cross check and verify my experiences of healing with those of others in the field. I am grateful to the many practitioners who have taken the trouble to pen their findings and published these. I have referred to many of their works as listed under the References section. I hope that this work adds to the body of knowledge available.

I owe a debt of gratitude to many people who have been of help, encouragement and motivation to write this book, especially Sujata Madhok, Rashme Sehgal, Nandini Mohan, Hardeep and Timmy Puri.

I have written this work to share my experiences of healing. I hope that my readers will find the work useful in their pursuit of health, wellness and happiness.

Inder Puri

Dedicated to the
Sanginis of the Air Force

Introduction

Seeing vast ailing masses of people crowding all departments of all hospitals compels one to ponder, is disease or injury inevitable sometimes in everyone's life? Is it inevitable that each one of us will be sick sometimes? Or, is it the fear of the unknown that impels us to seek medical intervention at the first sign of disease or distress? What thought do we give to OUR BODY, this wonderful, complicated, working on its own machine? Is the body designed to be dependent on outside intervention for survival? Or is it competent to take care of itself on its own?

Another thought. Are we alone in this word? When we look around we find that nature has provided a vast array of flora and fauna, besides us human beings. They are meant to exist and prosper within the laws of nature. How can we also not follow the rules of nature for our existence and wellbeing? Human existence and wellbeing may be regarded as a trinary entity of three components namely Body, Mind & Soul.

Human progress in all fields has created an environment of hard work (extremely long working hours), time bound, higher and higher targets and stiff competition that leads to flagrant flouting of nature's laws. It is all wilful. This overemphasis on work is to ensure a safe and secure future at the expense of the individual's health and goodwill. This leads to health problems affecting the body, mind and emotional wellbeing. Invariably an individual becomes a prisoner of the system. Caught in the quagmire, he begins taking short cuts to sustain and thrive. If only a person can take out some time for himself and undertake steps to strengthen his SELF for his own wellbeing.

Having been exposed to the ancient (recently revived) alternate systems of Healing and Magnetic Therapy for over twenty years, I am compelled to give some thought to the aspects of preventing ailments for the wellbeing of individuals and society.

Foremost, it must not be taken for granted that our body system will continue working optimally all the time irrespective of our lifestyle and indiscriminate flouting of natural laws. Just ponder, how much time do we give to ourselves? Do we ever give a thought to what keeps us going? How conversant are we with the functioning of our body? Does the body work independently? Or, is there any interconnection between the different parts of the body—do limbs/organs have support from other parts of the body?

Foremost it must be stated that the common denominator in all the alternate systems of healing is the belief that a specific pattern of electric energy is flowing all the time in our bodies. As long as this energy flows we are alive and kicking. This energy is called by different names around the world, e.g. in India it is known as 'Prana', in China it is known as 'Chi', in Japan it is 'Qui' and in Russia it is 'Blood Plasma'.

All alternate systems recognize that ailments occur when there is a disruption in the flow of energy. So, to regain health and wellbeing it is imperative that we try to remove the disruption and ensure uninterrupted flow of energy.

According to the principles of five phases, all things including the human body are divided into five elements represented by Fire (associated with heart and small intestine), Earth (associated with spleen and stomach), Sky/Aakash (associated with lung and large intestine), Water (associated with kidney and bladder), Air (associated with liver and gall bladder). The Chinese experts have two changes in the five phases, namely, Wood in place of Air and Metal in place of Aakash. Since these five elements are regarded as energetic qualities inherent in all things, their inter-relationship is due the existence of two cycles, namely the Generating Cycle and the Controlling Cycle.

The flow of energy in the body is through 14 meridians which cover the entire body. Six meridians have their start/end points on the hands, six meridians have their start/end points on the feet. Two central meridians (one in front of the body and one on the back) end on the face. One starts from a point between the anus and the genitalia. The other starts at a point between the anus and coccyx.

The principles of the therapies are closely linked to the concept of YIN-YANG. Though they may appear to be only symbols and many call them antiquated and unscientific, the concept embodied by YIN-YANG is timeless. YIN and YANG are two complementary opposites. YIN represents the aspects of quiescence and YANG the aspect of activity. Almost everything can be divided into YIN and YANG. What needs emphasis is that YIN and YANG while being two opposites are NOT two separate entities. Both can be found in the same place, like the two sides of a coin. Viewed from one side it is YIN and viewed from the other side it is YANG. They co-exist in the same sphere.

Whenever there is a deficiency in any one meridian, there is a need for tonification in the related meridian to restore the balance. If there is excess energy in any meridian it requires to be dispersed. The method employed is to apply pressure (either with hands or a gadget) to the points to restore the balance. Like acupressure, Magnetic Therapy is another ancient system which has been used in all parts of the globe since the past 2500 years. Magnets were found, recognized and used in Europe, Africa and Asia. In Greece Magnets were called Magnetis or 'Magneseto', in England the term was 'lodestone', in France it was 'Aimant', in India it was 'Chumbak; in China it was 'Chusi' and in Urdu and Persian it was 'Magnetees'.

Magnetism is the basic principle that dominates and governs the infinite universe and holds the various heavenly bodies in natural bondage. The earth, moon, sun and the other planets in our galaxy transmit their own magnetic emanations which greatly influence our lives. There are various schools of thought about the source of magnetism on earth. But what has been established is that the earth is a huge natural magnet.

The human body itself is a magnet. It is governed by the natural laws and actions and deeds done in natural ways give peace and pacification. Magnets have been successfully used to treat human diseases. Magnetised water is used in many countries as it is found to act against various diseases and help maintain good health. Its anti-ageing properties have also been recognized.

Good health is the noblest gift of god. According to W.H.O. good health is described as 'A state of complete physical and mental social wellbeing and not merely the absence of disease or infirmity.' Medical science can prevent and cure illness but it cannot ensure good health. Good health is dependent not on the services available but on one's SELF.

Man cannot run away from disease creeping into his physical self. But he can create internal and external safeguards against any impending illness. Safeguarding requires increasing resistance in the body by:

(a) Cleansing the body of any undesirable accumulations, removing obstacles and regularizing working of the human machinery.

(b) Providing new vigour and stimulation to the energies in the body.

Magnets are capable of accomplishing the above two objectives.

There is a great similarity in the approach of Alternative Systems like Acupressure and Magnetic Therapy as both systems work through outward application on various parts of the body without any internal medication. It has been established that application of Magnets on various Acupressure points gives beneficial results. A combination of the two therapies can increase the beneficial effects manifold.

While each of the above aspects has been elaborated in later chapters, a brief insight into the two therapies i.e. Acupressure and Magnetic Therapy would help clarify the efficacy of the two systems.

The laws of nature clearly point to the following essentials for good health:

(a) Self Awareness.

(b) Proper and regulated Breathing.

(c) Proper Diet.

(d) Proper Elimination.

(e) Proper Sleep.

(f) Proper Exercise.

(g) Proper Sex.

This book is aimed at making the average individual aware of the functioning of the body. It is designed to give a glimpse of the laws of nature and why it is necessary to follow them to the extent possible to experience the joys and happiness of a healthy mind, body and soul.

Contents

CHAPTER 1

Insight into Acupressure

Acupressure is drugless alternative therapy which:

(a) Has a holistic approach.

(b) Is totally non-invasive.

(c) Combines diagnostic and curative methods.

(d) Has the same approach for both cure and prevention of ailments.

Basic Premise

(a) Energy flows in our body as long as we are alive.

(b) It flows along 14 channels known as Meridians.

(b) Some Meridians are YIN (Negative force) and some YANG (Positive Force).

(d) The balance and harmony between YIN and YANG meridians indicates ALL IS WELL and one is healthy.

(e) The ailments occur when there is an imbalance in any meridian.

(f) Emphasis is laid on removing the imbalance to heal the ailment.

What are YIN and YANG?

(a) They are expressions of two complementary opposites.

(b) YIN represents quiescence (Resting State) and YANG represents activity. They are like two sides of a coin which coexist within the same sphere.

YIN and YANG in the Human Body

(a)   The lower half is YIN and the upper half is YANG

(b)   The front of the body is YIN and the back is YANG.

(c)   Dense Organs are YIN and Hollow Organs are YANG.

(d)   The YIN Organs are:
   (i)   Heart
   (ii)   Heart Pericardium
   (iii)   Lungs
   (iv)   Spleen
   (v)   Liver
   (vi)   Kidneys (it is the most YIN)

(e)   The YANG Organs are:
   (i)   Large Intestine
   (ii)   Stomach
   (iii)   Bladder
   (iv)   Small Intestine
   (v)   Triple Warmer (energy flow in nerves)
   (vi)   Gall Bladder

Meridians that govern other meridians:

(i)   Governing Vessel (at the back of the body including the spine)

(ii)   Conception Vessel (at the front of the body

Meridians on the Hands

A.   **Lung Meridian** – has 11 points:

(i)   Starts at point medial to the coracoids process.

(ii)   Ends at radial side of thumbnail

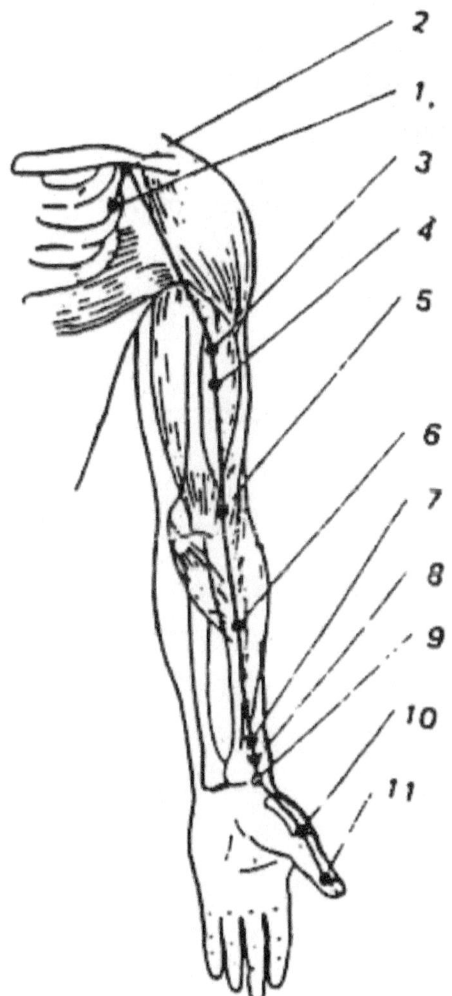

Important points

1. Lung 5—located at 2" above the volar wrist crease 1½"above the radialstyloid process.

2. Lung 7—It is a master point and very effective for pulmonary diseases such as oedema, pneumonia, bronchitis, asthma, headache.

3. Lung 9—located at the radial aspect of the volar wrist crease. It influences the strength and tone of several shoulder muscles for treatment of bronchitis, cough, asthma and addiction to nicotine (smoking).

B.   Large Intestine—It has 20 points

(i)   Starts at radial side of index finger

(ii) Ends at Nasolobial fold

Generally used to treat:

(i)   Head, Neck and Shoulder pain.

(ii) Gastrointestinal problems.

(iii) Nasal Congestion.

(iv) Toothache.

(v)   Dermatological Conditions.

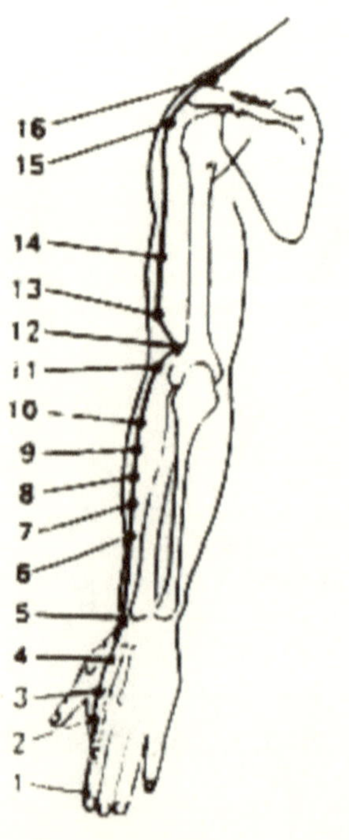

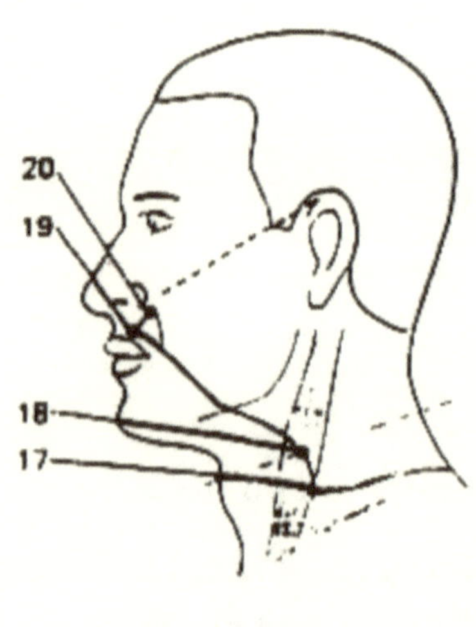

Important Points

I. **Large Intestine 4** (near the junction of the thumb and index finger metacarpal bones). It is a master point—effective for Head conditions: Cold, flu, headaches, upper extremity pain, allergies, dermatologic conditions, hypoglycaemia and addiction to smoking.

II. **Large Intestine 11** (at the lateral elbow crease). Effective for elbow problems, high blood pressure, torticollis, acne, rashes and colon problems.

C. Heart Pericardium – It has 9 points.

It starts at 1" lateral to the left nipple and ends at radial side of third fingernail. Generally used for treating:

(a) Cardiac Conditions such as angina, arrhythmias.

(b) Inter Costal neuralgia.

(c) Rib and Chest pain.

(d) Diaphragmatic Spasms.

(e) Pulmonary Diseases.

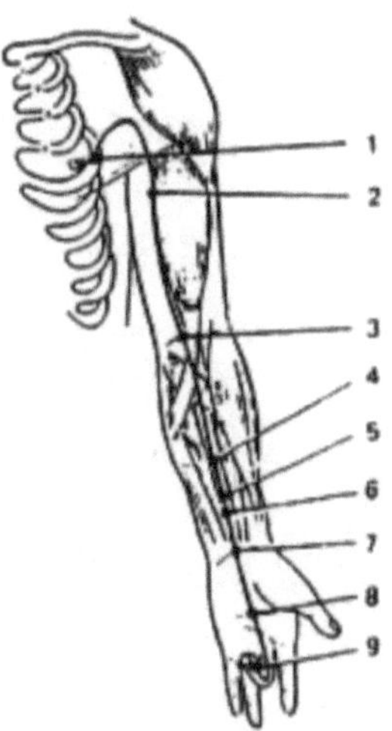

Important points:

1. HC -3 (in the cubital crease of the ulnar side of the bicep tendon). Angina, rheumatic heart disease, myocarditis, palpitations, gastroenteritis, elbow pain.

2. HC-6 (2" above transverse wrist crease between Palmaris longus and flexor carpi radialis tendons) cardiac heart failure, rheumatic heart disease, gastrointestinal problems, indigestion, nausea, vomiting, gravidarum, hyperthyroidism, painful throat, diaphragmatic spasms, migraine, dizziness.

3. HC-8 (with fist clenched, the point is in the centre of the palm between the second and the third finger) Dupuytrens contracture, acne, coma, shock, diaphragmatic spasms.

D. Triple Warmer

It has 23 points, starts at ulnar side of fourth finger and ends at lateral eyebrow.

Generally used for:

Autonomic nervous system balance. Ear conditions such as deafness and tinnitus.

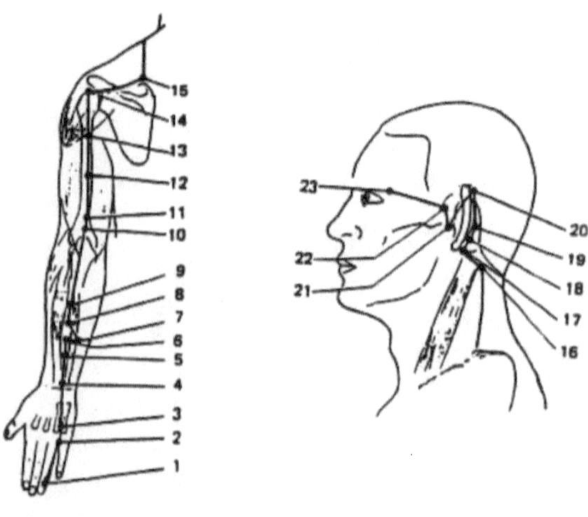

Important points

(a) TW 3 (on dorsum of hand behind the metacarpal phalangeal joint between 4th and 5th metacarpal)—for ear disorders temporal headache and shoulder pain.

(b) TW 5 (2" above the dorsal wrist crease between the ulna and radial bones)—for balancing automatic nervous system, ear disorders, gout, arthritis, and migraine.

(c) TW 10 (1" above olecranon when elbow is flexed)—for neck and shoulder pain, tonsillitis, migraine.

(d) TW 17 (behind the earlobe in the styloid depression)—useful for ear disorders, paralysis, Bells palsy, eye diseases, cataract.

(e) TW 23 (in a small depression near the lateral edge of the eyebrow)—useful for eye diseases, blurred vision, headache.

E. Heart Meridian

It has 9 points. Starts at axilla of axillary artery. Ends at radial side of the fifth finger at the fingernail.

Used for:

(a) Cardiac conditions such as palpitation, angina, arrhythmias.

(b) Forgetfulness, Alzheimers.

(c) Hypertension.

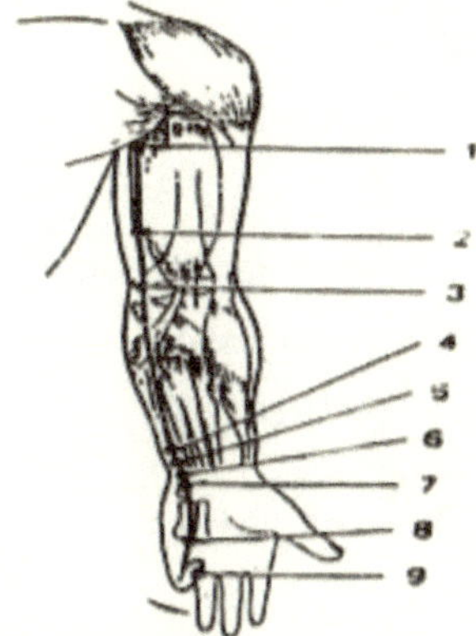

Important points

(a) H-3 (with elbow bend lies in depression between the medial condyle of the humerus and the end of cubital crease). Cardiac conditions, anxiety, headache, dizziness, chest pain, elbow pain.

(b) H-5 (1" above H-7 on the ulnar side of the volar surface of the forearm). Chest pain, angina, dizziness, headaches.

(c) H-7 (at ulnar aspect of the volar wrist crease in the depression at the ulna side of the pisiform bone). Angina, arrhythmia, anxiety, heart diseases, oedema, fever, nervousness, irritability, insomnia, bronchitis, smoking addiction, nausea, vomiting.

(d) H-8 (with the hand clenched, point lies on the palm between the 4th and 5th fingers).Rheumaticheart disease, angina, arrhythmia, palpitation.

(e) H-9 (on the radial side of the 5th finger nail). In case of cardiac problems, press the little fingernail and rotate it round and round four to five times. Repeat twice.

F. Small Intestine Meridian

It has 19 points. Starts at ulnar side of little fingernail. Ends in front of tragus.

Useful for:

(i) Ear conditions such as otitis media, hearing disorders, tinnitus.

(ii) Arthritis.

Important points

(i) S1-3 (with clenched fist, point lies in a depression at the end of crease by the head of 5th metacarpal bone). Low back pain, arthritis, gout, tinnitus, deafness, stiff neck.

(ii) S1-6 (with forearm and palm facing the chest, point lies in a depression on the radial side of the ulnar head). Stiff neck, low back pain, eye disorders and arthritis of the upper extremities.

(iii) S1-19 (in front of and at the middle of the tragus (in a depression, when mouth is open). Deafness tinnitus, ear infection, facial paralysis.

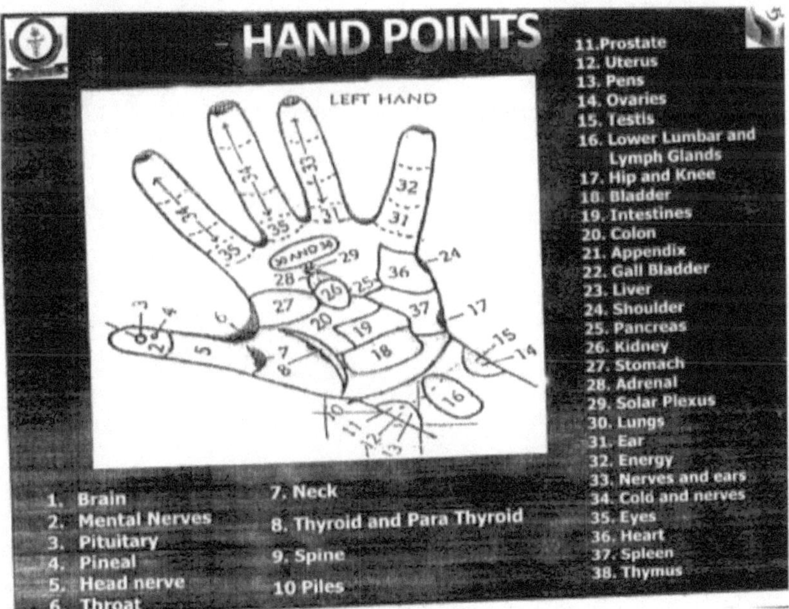

Meridians on the Feet

A. Spleen: It has 21 points

Starts at medial side of first toenail. Ends at sixth intercostal space.

Useful for:

(i) Gynaecological conditions.

(ii) Urinary problems.

(iii) Hematological problems.

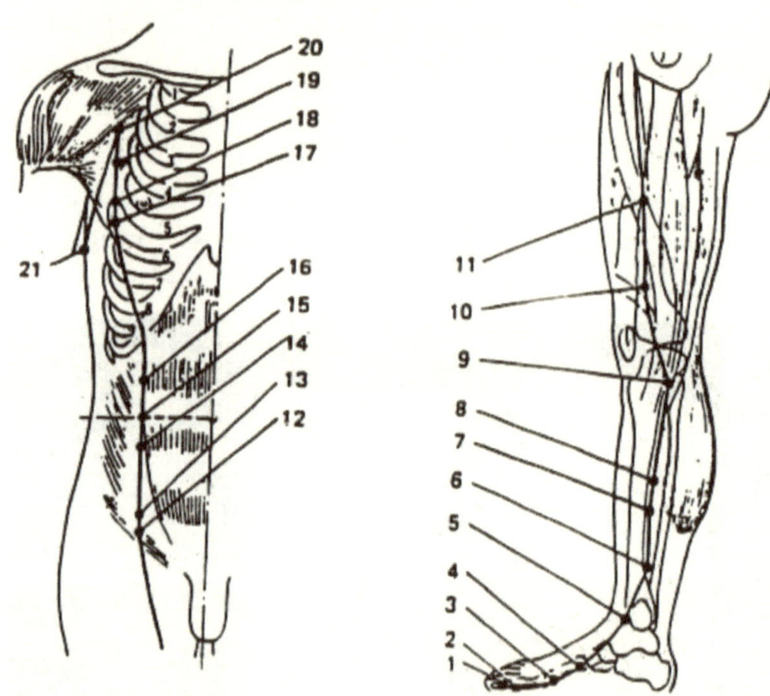

Important points

(i) Sp-4 (on the medial aspect at the proximal end of the first metatarsal bone). Digestive problems, hypoglycaemia, gravidarum.

(ii) Sp-6 (3" above the medial malleolus on the posterior border of the tibia). Reproductive problems, impotency, female sterility, incontinence, dysuria, oedema, abdominal distention, hypoglycaemia, diabetes.

(iii) Sp-9 (approx. 2" above the superior border of the patella on the medial thigh). Knee pain, menstrual problems, impotency, frequent urination, arthritis.

(iv) Sp-10 (approx. 2" above the superior border of the patella on the medial thigh). Knee pain, menstrual problems, allergies, urticaria.

B. Liver

It has 14 points.

(i) Starts at the lateral side of the first toe.

(ii) Anterolateral abdominal wall.

Useful for:

(a) Digestive disorders.
(b) Biliary diseases.
(c) Impotency.
(d) Detoxification.

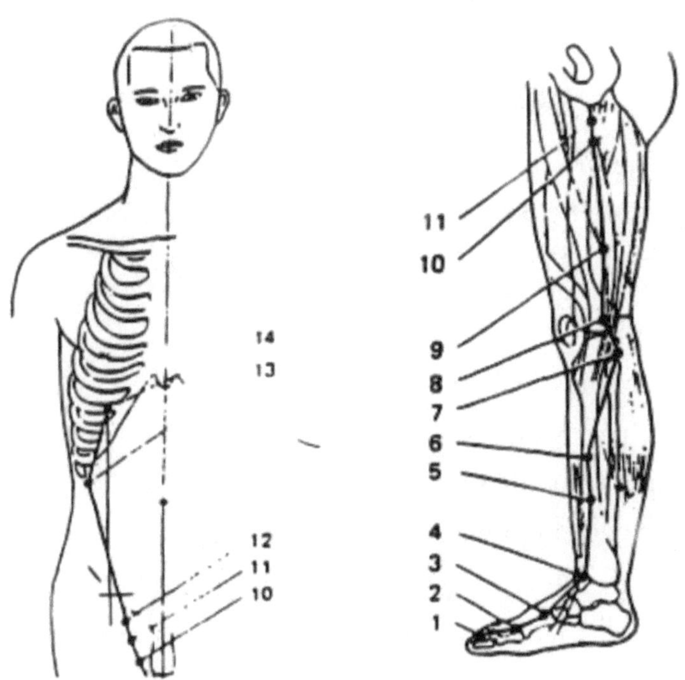

Important points

(a) LV-2 (in the web between the 1st and 2nd toes). Red swollen eyes, glaucoma, urogenital problems, arthritis, enuresis, orchitis, penile pain, hypertension, gout, oedema, urticaria.

(b) LV-3 (2" above LV-2 between 1st and 2nd metatarsals). Head conditions, migraine, headaches, dizziness, insomnia, epilepsy, allergies, leukaemia, hypertension, detoxification, drug abuse, alcoholism, addiction to smoking.

(c) LV-5 (3" above medial malleolus at the posterior border of the tibia bone). Urogenital problems, dysuria, irregular menses, impotency, orchitis.

(d) LV-8 (in a depression at the junction of the semitendinous and semimembranosus tendons of the medial aspect of the popliteal fossa). Dysuria, impotency, penis pain, spermatorrhea, prostate disease and knee pain.

C. Stomach Meridian

It has 45 points

    (i) **Starting point:** Superior to infra-orbital foramen

    (ii) **Ending Point:** Lateral side of second toenail.

Useful for:

(a) Gastro-intestinal problems.

(b) Facial paralysis.

(c) Temporal mandibular joint pain.

(d) Systematic improvement of muscle tone.

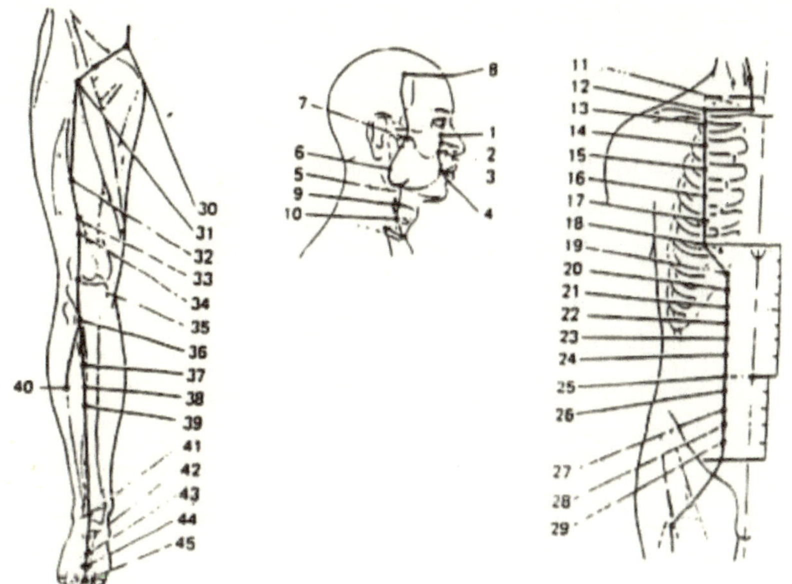

Important points

(a) St2 (at infraorbital foramen on a line with the centre of eye pupil). Nerve paralysis, facial palsy, maxillary sinusitis, eye conditions, rhinitis.

(b) St4 (at corner of mouth). Facial palsy, trigeminal neuralgia.

(c) St7 (in the mandibular notch). Temporomandibular joint problems, trigeminal neuralgia, toothache.

(d) St25 (approx. 2" lateral to the umbilicus). Abdominal distress, diverticulitis constipation, insomnia, menstrual problems.

(e) St36 (in a depression on the anterolateral leg between the tibial tuberosity and head of fibula). General muscle tone, infections, anaemia, abdominal pain, colon diseases, hypertension.

D. Gall Bladder Meridian

It has 44 points

    (i) Starts at approx. ½" posterior to lateral canthus of eye.

    (ii) Ends at lateral side of 4th toenail.

    Useful for:

    (a) Pain along lateral side of body.

    (b) Biliary disorders

    (c) Headaches

    (d) Deafness

    (e) Tinnitus

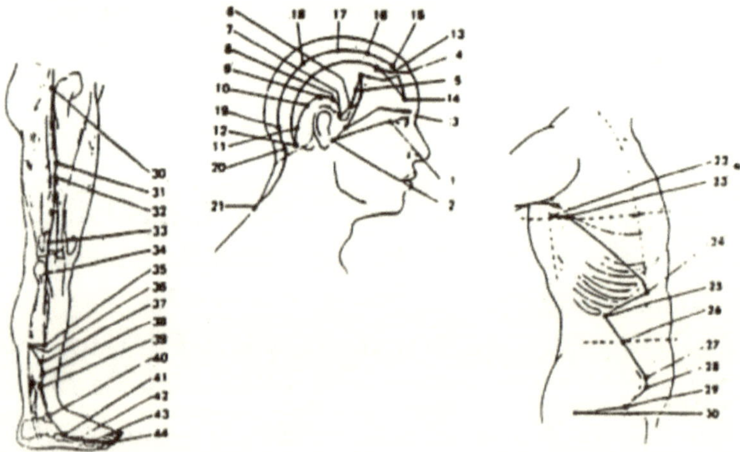

Important points

(a) GB-1 (1/2" lateral to the lateral canthus of the eye). Glaucoma, optic nerve atrophy, headache, facial palsy.

(b) GB-2 (in front of and at lower end of tragus when mouth is open). Deafness, tinnitus, otitis media, facial palsy, parotiditis, toothache.

(c) GB-14 (1" above eyebrow in line with centre of pupil). Headache, facial palsy, eye disease.

(d) GB-20 (in a depression at base of skull between SCM and trapezius muscles). Headache, stiff neck, rhinitis, common cold, sinusitis, deafness, tinnitus.

(e) GB-26 (midaxilliary line on a level with the umbilicus.

(f) GB-30 (approximately one third of the distance between the greater trochocentre of the femur). Low back pain, sciatica, arthritis of hip joint.

(g) GB-34 (anterior to and slightly below the head of the fibula bone). Gall bladder disease, digestive problems, constipation, stress, enuresis, knee or leg pain, weak legs, pain of shoulder, hypertension.

E. Bladder Meridian

It has 67 points

(i) Starts at Medial Canthus of the eye

(ii) Ends at lateral side of fifth toenail

Useful for:

(a) Posterior pain

(b) Headaches

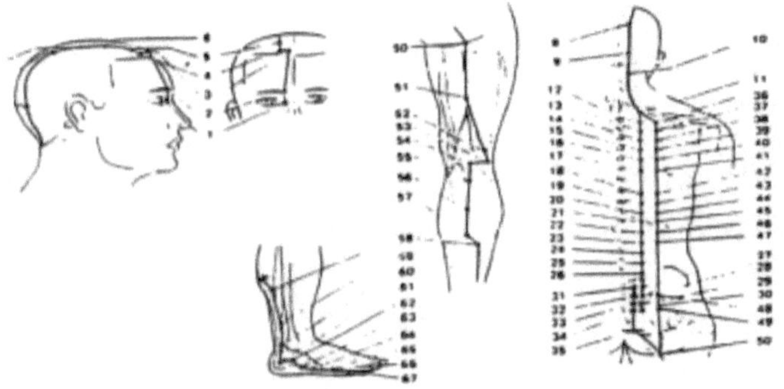

Important points

(a) BL-1 (1" above the medial canthus of the eye). Cataract, optic nerve atrophy, glaucoma, conjunctivitis.

(b) BL-2 (In the eyebrow at the medial end). Headache, facial paralysis, eye diseases.

(c) BL-10 (in a depression lateral to midline of occiput). Occipital headaches, stiff neck, migraines.

(d) BL-13 (1.5" lateral to T-3). Common cold, cough, bronchitis, headache, asthma.

(e) BL-20 (1.5"lateral to T-11). Gastritis, anaemia, indigestion, abdominal distention, ulcers.

(f) BL-25 (1.5" lateral to lumber-4). Low back pain, sacroiliac pain, dysentery, constipation.

(g) BL-50 (mid-point of buttock crease). Low back pain, sciatica, constipation, haemorrhoids.

(h) BL-54 (in the middle of the popliteal fossa). Low back pain, sciatica, knee or leg pain.

(i) BL-60 (midway between lateral malleolus and Achilles tendon). Sciatica, low back pain, knee, leg and ankle pain, Mortons neuroma.

F. Kidney Meridian

It has 27 points

Starts at plantar surface of the foot between 2nd and 3rd metatarsal bones. Ends at junction of the clavicle and first rib at sternum.

Useful for:

(a) Fluid imbalance

(b) Urinary problems

(c) Impotency

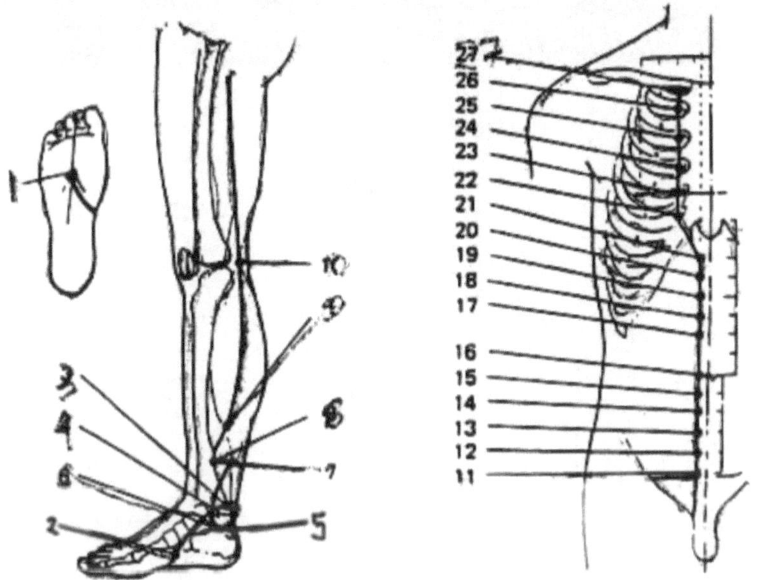

Important points

(a) K-2 (in a depression below the navicular bone tubercle, inferior and anterior to medial malleolus). Cystitis, enuresis, diabetes, irregular menses, female sterility.

(b) K-3 (midway between medial malleolus and Achilles tendon). Enuresis, cystitis nephritis, impotency, ankle pain, alopecia, diabetes, leukaemia.

(c) K-7 (2" above medial malleolus). Enuresis, cystitis, nephritis, orchitis, diabetes, herpes.

(d) K-10 (at medial end of popliteal crease between semimembranosus and semitendinosus tendons). Knee arthritis or knee pain, urogenital troubles.

(e) K-15 (1" below and 1.5" lateral to the umbilicus). Abdominal pain, constipation (at the medial end of the clavicle at the sternum). Cough, bronchitis, asthma, chest pain.

FEET POINTS

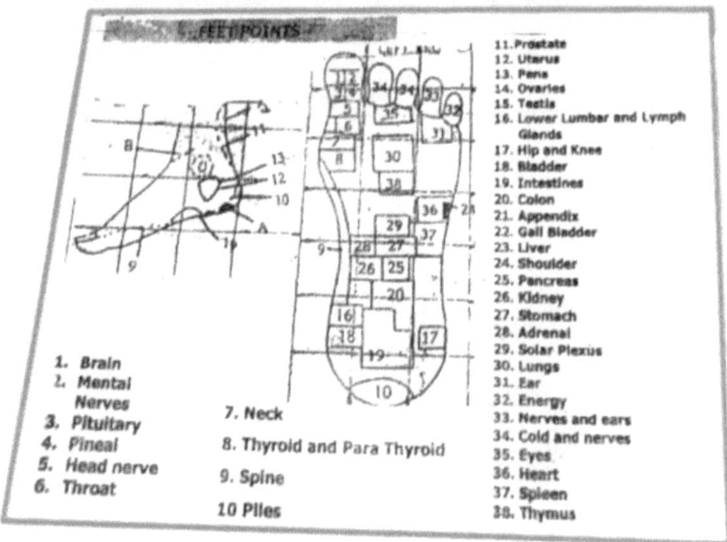

The Two Central Meridians

A. Conception Vessel (CV) Meridians

It has 24 points

(i) Starts at perineum between the anus and the genitalia.

(ii) Ends just below lower hip.

Useful for:

(a) Anterior pain

(b) Impotency

(c) Irregular or painful menses

(d) Gastric pain

(e) Enuresis

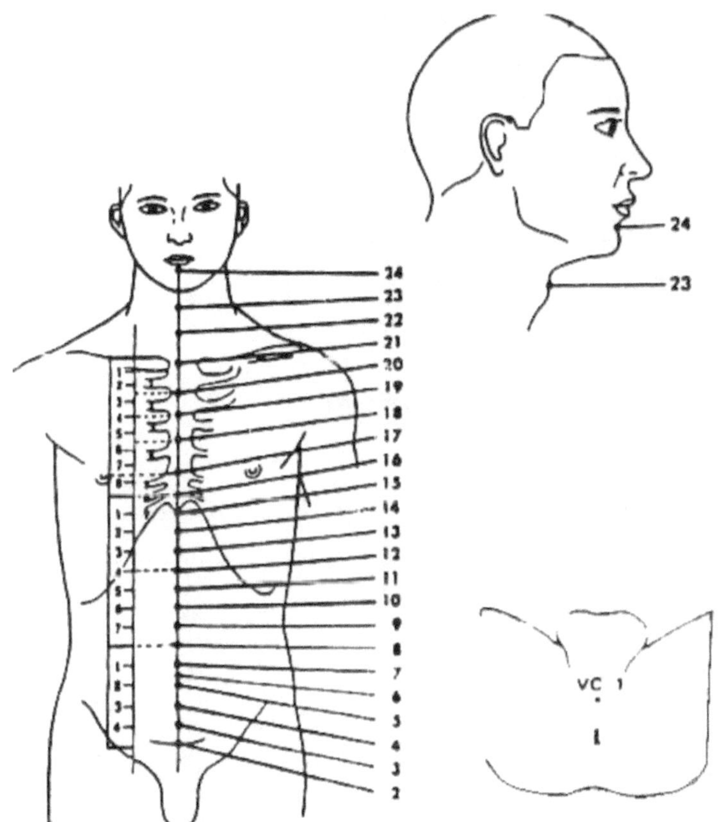

Important points

(a) CV-3 (midline 4" below the umbilicus). Enuresis, incontinence, impotency, irregular menses, dysmenorrhea, female sterility, menopause, sciatica.

(b) CV-4 (midline 4" below the umbilicus). General weakness, gastro intestinal pain, urogenital infection, impotency, hot flushes, hypoglycaemia, low back pain, sciatica.

(c) CV-6 (midline 1.5" below Umbilicus). Dysmenorrhea, irregular menses, hot flushes, impotency, incontinence, ulcer, abdominal pain.

(d) CV-12 (midline 4" above the Umbilicus). Ulcer, gastritis, diarrhoea, constipation, hypoglycaemia.

(e) CV-17 (midline between the nipples). Asthma, bronchitis, chest pain, mastitis, insufficient lactation, cardiac disease.

(f) CV-22 (in depression at the suprasternal fossa). Throat and lung troubles, asthma, bronchitis, pharyngitis, laryngitis, goitre, thyroid disease, diseases of the vocal cord.

B. Governing Vessel (GV) Meridian

It has 28 points.

(i) Starts at: perineum between the anus and tip of coccyx.

(ii) Ends at frenulum between the upper lip and the gum).

Useful for:

(a) Endocrine imbalance.
(b) Back pain.
(c) Spinal pain
(d) Pelvic disorder

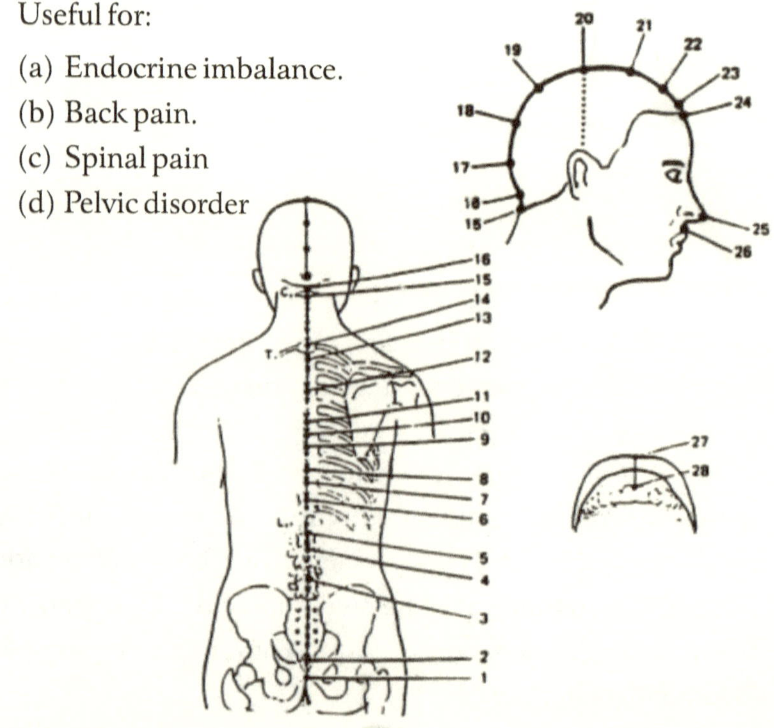

Important points

(a) GV-3 (between 4th and 5th lumbar spinous process). Low back pain, diarrhoea, irregular menses, impotency.

(b) GV-14 (between 7th cervical and 1st thoracic spinous process). Psychoses, seizures, asthma, bronchitis, emphysema, colds, posterior shoulder pain

(c) GV-20 (at the vertex of head on a line drawn from the ear tips). Head conditions, stress, nasal congestion, insomnia, headache, seizures, tinnitus, allergic rhinitis

(d) GV-23 (1" posterior to hairline from the forehead). Headache, rhinitis, nasal congestion, sore eyes, keratitis.

(e) GV-25 (in the tip of nose). Shock, hypertension, nose bleed, rhinitis, hangover.

(f) GV-26 (in the philtrum 1/3 of the distance down from the nose) shock, coma, seizures, nausea, eye or mouth infections, facial oedema.

MERIDIAN POINTS ON THE FACE

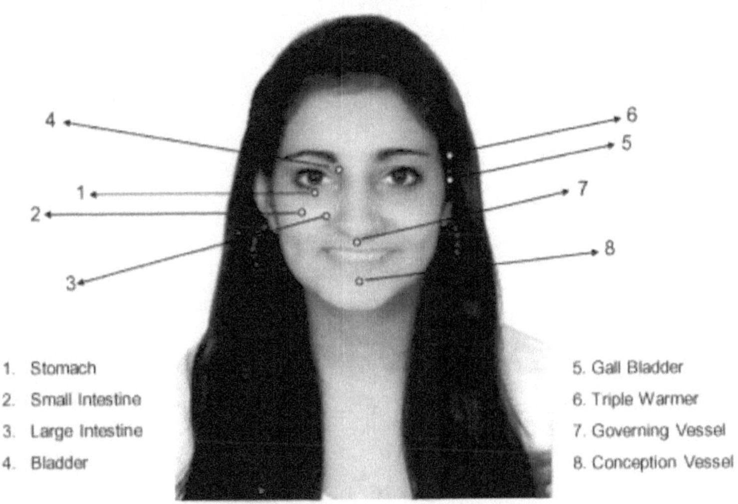

1. Stomach	5. Gall Bladder
2. Small Intestine	6. Triple Warmer
3. Large Intestine	7. Governing Vessel
4. Bladder	8. Conception Vessel

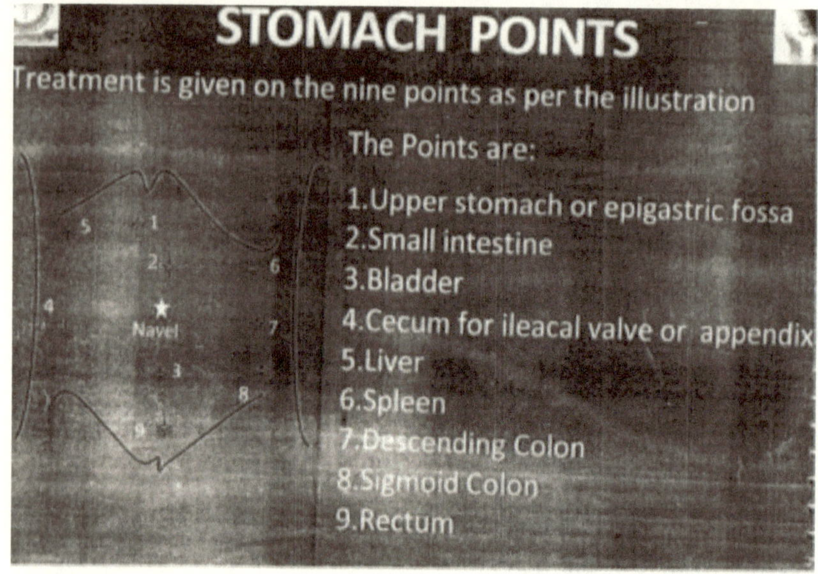

Useful for:

1. Judging state of stomach
2. Help in digestion
3. Prevent onset of ailments

CHAPTER 2

Elements Constituting the Body

FIRE—Heart Pericardium, Small Intestine, Triple Warmer
EARTH—Stomach and Spleen
METAL—Lung and Large Intestine
WATER—Bladder and Kidney
WOOD—Gall Bladder and Liver

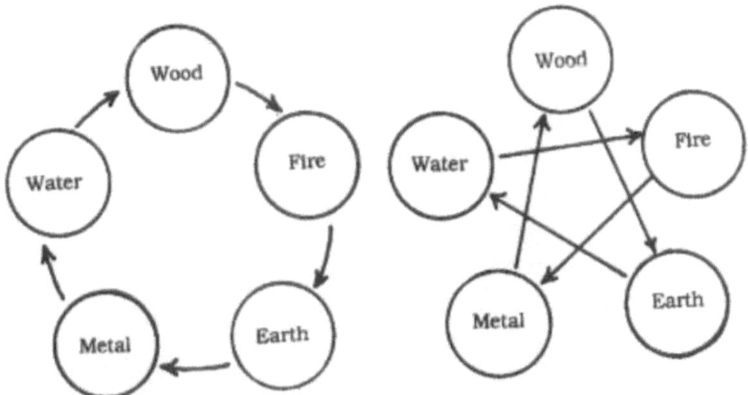

The energy that flows to and from the brain controls billions of brain cells which are found to be of five types, representing the basic elements that the human body consists of, namely, earth, water, fire, air and space. According to Chinese philosophy, metal and wood substitute air and space.

The principle of the five elements is accepted in acupressure and the elements are represented by the fingers of the body.

Since there are parts of ONE body, they have a method of controlling and also helping one another to ensure a perfect balance of the elements. Any imbalance created by disturbance (excess or less) of any one element leads to imbalance in other elements and this becomes the root cause of an ailment.

The two cycles which connect the elements are:

(a) Productive Cycle – in this cycle excess in one element (say earth) leads to deficiency in the next element (metal, in this case). Thus elements try to keep the next one in line supplied of energy.

(b) Controlling Cycle – in this relationship, the elements have the power and capacity to control other elements. For example, water douses fire and earth gives water.

CHAPTER 3

Endocrine Glands

There is more to the human body than the physical body itself. Most people consider the physical body and material world to be the only reality that exists. These are perhaps the only things that can be discerned with our physical senses. Besides the numerous bodies within and around the human body there is a complex energy system at work without which the body could not exist.

This energy system comprising of energy centers and energy channels is known by different names. The ancient Indians called it Chakras (Energy Centers and Ida/pingala energy channels).

In both the allopathic and some alternate systems of medicine these are referred to as endocrine glands. The endocrine gland system forms a vital part in alternate therapies like acupressure, sujok, reflexology, reiki and magnetic therapy etc. These glands secrete a variety of hormones directly into the blood thereby preserving chemical balance and connections amongst the internal organs. They control the MENTAL, PHYSICAL and EMOTIONAL well being of every living human being. They are body regulators and protectors. I give them due importance by mentioning them first, as their balance ensures total well being of every human. They are SEVEN in number. They are interrelated and dependent on one another and assist each other in proper functioning, following the holistic approach. All treatments in alternate systems should start with balancing of these glands irrespective of ailments.

The main function of these glands is control of the five basic elements of the body. The functions include:

A. Control of 5 basic elements of the body.

B. Adjust the body to the changing environment and protect against illness.

C. Play a vital role in the development of our body and mind and also in the development of our looks and even character.

The location of these glands is placed herewith:

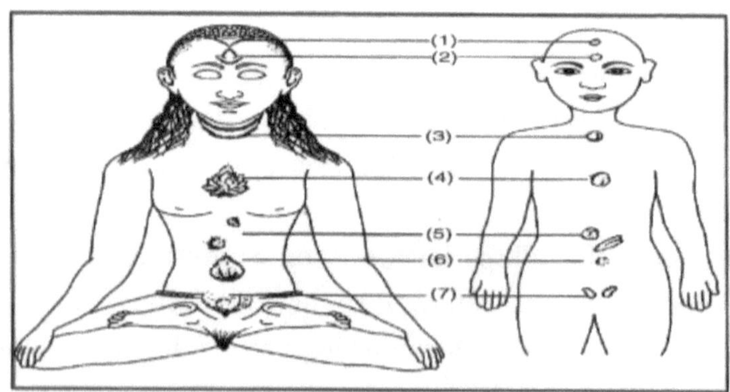

1. Pineal gland 2. Pituitary 3. Thyroid, para-thyroid 4. Thymus 5. Adrenal and Pancreas 6. Solar Plexus 7. Sex/Gonad glands.

Some information about these glands, starting from the base of the body:

Sex Glands

(a) **Location:** These are located under the tail bone between the coccyx and perineum below the anus.

(b) **Functions**: (i) Maintain an unbroken chain of procreation.

(ii) Regulate the water elements and also nerves, cells, flesh, bones, bone marrow and semen.

(iii) Regulate the digestion of phosphorous in the body, thus regulating the heat within the body.

(b) If the functioning of the gland is predominant: (i) Life is filled with satisfaction, stability and inner strength.

(ii) Actions guided by desire to be creative

(c) In case of disharmonious functioning: (i) Thoughts and actions revolve around material possessions and security.

(ii) Overindulgence in sensual pleasures such as good food, alcohol and sex.

(iii) Boys tend to self abuse, masturbate, have erotic dreams and become shy.

(iv) The growth of the body is affected and beard appears prematurely.

(v) Root cause of inability to bear a child.

(vi) Main cause of weight gain in females after delivery or sterilization.

(vii) Insufficient working causes complications during menopause.

(viii) Malfunctioning noticeable when children are getting mature (12-15 years). Girls have menstrual problems (late, painful or scanty) leading to pimples and excess heat in the body. Too much of bleeding causes anemia. Some may have excess hair on the face and underdeveloped growth of the body.

(ix) Feelings of rage, anger, violence indicating lack of trust.

(x) Feelings of uncertainty and insecurity.

Solar Plexus Glands

(a) **Location:** Halfway between the pubic bone and navel situated on top of each kidney.

(b) **Body association:** Pelvic girdle, kidneys, spleen, liver, bladder and gall bladder and all liquids such as blood lymph, bile, gastric juice, sperm and regulation of the female cycle.

(c) **Harmonious functions of the Gland:** (i) Keenness of perception, tireless activities, inner energy and courage.

(ii) Helps proper oxygenation.

(iii) Develops organizing power.

(iv) Character building of a child.

(v) Regulates blood sugar levels.

(d) **In case of Disharmonious functioning:** (i) Abuse of natural vigour to satisfy lust or anti social activity.

(ii) Suffer a sense of vainglory and become conceited.

(iii) Become restless, impatient and short-tempered.

(iv) Not able to control diet and suffer from stomach ailments and blood pressure.

(v) Become fearful, timid, lose vigour to face problems of life.

Adrenal/Pancreas

(a) **Location:** Behind the stomach and lies transverse across the posterior abdominal wall at the level of $1^{st}/2^{nd}$ vertebrae.

(b) **Functions:** (i) Regulates digestion of sugar by creating insulin.

(ii) Without insulin the muscles are unable to use the sugar which circulates in the blood for energy.

(c) **Disharmonious functioning:** (i) If blood sugar is too high the excess is secreted by the kidneys and appears in the urine

(ii) If the islets of langerhans do not function properly there is lack of insulin resulting in diabetes.

(iii) Over-functioning of the glands leads to low BP and migraine and creates excess desire for sweet food and drinks.

Thymus Gland

(a) **Location:** In the thorax behind the sternum and in front of the heart.

(b) **Functions:** Consists mainly of lymphoid tissue and plays a part in the formation of lymphocytes.

(c) It protects the growing the child against disease.

(d) Plays an important role in keeping the body's immune system active.

(e) Once the body is developed this gland shrinks and stops its activities.

(f) In case it becomes active at a later age it produces dullness and general fatigue leading to total inactivity.

Thyroid/Parathyroid Glands

(a) **Location:** Between the depression in the neck and the larynx beginning at the cervical vertebra. The thyroid gland comprises two lobes which are situated on either side of the trachea and are joined together by an isthmus which passes in front of the trachea. There are four parathyroid glands, each one above the four poles of the thyroid gland.

(b) **Functions:** Controls air and lungs, regulates body temperature, governs energy production through control of calcium.

(c) **Hormones secreted**: Thyroxin and tridothyronine. These control iodine metabolism and the balance of calcium in our blood and tissues.

Harmonious Functioning: (a) Able to express feelings, thoughts and inner knowledge without fear.

(b) Able to express yourself with entire personality and at the same time remain silent and listen to others with all your heart and understanding.

(c) Speech is imaginative and perfectly clear and your voice is full and melodious.

(d) Not swayed by people's opinions.

(e) Able to maintain your independence, freedom and self-determination.

(f) Helps in concentration and balanced temperament and purity of heart, unselfishness.

Disharmonious Functioning: (a) In infancy hypothyroidism causes stunted growth and failure of mental development.

(b) In adults hypothyroidism causes obesity, dry skin and scanty hair. The metabolic rate is slowed down, causing difficulty in keeping warm, also leads to physical fatigue and asthma.

(c) Hyperthyroidism is associated with goitre. It leads to weakness, twisting of muscles, rickets, convulsions and development of children is retarded.

(d) Children become dull and fat. Symptoms include overgrowth, bulging eyes and protruding Adams Apple.

(e) The tone of voice may be noisy and the language may be unpleasant or cold and businesslike. The voice is loud but the words lack depth of meaning.

(f) The person tends to appear strong and does not permit himself to show any weakness.

(g) There is a tendency to attract attention to oneself.

(h) Body temperature remains high.

(i) Gets easily irritated.

Pineal Gland

(a) **Location:** Between the undersurface of the cerebrum and the mid brain in front of the cerebellum. It is small, reddish gray and of the size of a pea. Its main secretion is melatonin.

(b) **Functioning:** (a) Acts as organiser and controller of all glands.

(b) Regulates water balance in the body.

(c) Controls cerebral spinal fluid and sexual desire.

(d) Stimulates nerves.

(e) Affects the biological clock of the body.

If predominant:

(a) Generates a sense of sublimity, great wisdom and tenderness of heart.

(b) Not affected by physical sufferings and sorrows.

In case of any malfunction:

(a) Excess retention of fluid in the body.

(b) Tension and worry affect gland adversely.

(c) Leads to high blood pressure.

(d) Disturbs other glands and the digestive system.

(e) Awakens sex glands prematurely and even causes sexual delinquency.

Pituitary Gland

(a) **Location:** The king of all glands is located at the base of the brain and is about one 1 cm in diameter and consists of an anterior and posterior lobe.

(b) **Functioning:** (a) Controls the elements of air and space.

(b) Ensures proper functioning of all glands, even rectifies their faults.

(c) Controls brain power and memory, will power, sight, hearing and sense of discrimination.

(d) If predominant, people become geniuses in their chosen fields.

In case of malfunctioning:

(a) People become top heavy i.e. they live completely in the mental sphere.

(b) Life determined exclusively by reason and intellect, can fall prey to intellectual arrogance.

(c) Actions may tend to feed ego.

(d) Life dominated by materialistic desires and physical needs.

(e) Lose temper in demanding situations.

(f) People become pitiless, bullies and criminals.

(g) Main cause of weight gain in women post childbirth.

(h) Gland could get damaged due to fear, injury or stress during pregnancy. This could lead to malfunctioning of other glands and even cause birth of retarded children. Some children could become mean, heartless, disobedient, mischievous bullies and liars.

(i) Less secretion causes excess urination and leads to diabetes.

(j) Overworking of gland during childhood makes children

big physically while insufficient functioning may result in stunted growth.

Exercise for Endocrine Glands

The aim of the exercise is to bring about balance in the glands. Irrespective of ailment related to any of the glands, all 7 points need to be pressed at one go each time. For maintaining balance and harmony these points need to be pressed on a regular basis. The method of pressing is:

(a) Press each point starting from the Pituitary on the thumb for 10 seconds thrice, with a gap of 3 seconds between each pressing action. The treatment on one hand would suffice for one time.

(b) Another way of putting pressure on these points is by using 'Kharaon' (a wooden slipper with wooden knob which is grasped between the big toe and the one next to it).

The major glands points are located on the front half of the foot. Walking a couple of steps would put adequate pressure on these points. Use of 'Kharaon' for 10 minutes would suffice to energise these points. The other glands on the ankles could be pressed by rubbing around the ankles 5 times (on both sides).

(c) The reflex point for the 'King of all Glands' the Pituitary is located on the palm side of the thumb and is the organiser and controller of the other glands. The reflex point for the Pineal gland is located next to it. For stimulation of the points I strongly recommend the regular use of a rosary or 'mala' (a string of 108 beads, commonly used for religious purposes). Roll each bead over the centre of the thumb up to the top phalanx. It may take 3-4 minutes to roll all the 108 beads. A 'Mala' can be used any time without any restriction.

Chapter 4

Brief Insight into Magnetic Therapy

Basic Premise

- There is a magnetic field in our body at all times.
- Each organ has a separate magnetic field of varying intensity.
- When there is a disruption in the magnetic field of any organ, ailment occurs.
- Magnets can be used effectively by placing them on specific pain points as identified by the Acupressure System.

Basic Facts

- Each magnet has two sides, the North Pole and the South Pole.
- North Pole (Red colour side of magnets) stimulates and promotes healing, growth and activity.
- South Pole (Blue colour side of magnets generally used) calms, sedates, reduces inflammation and pain and promotes healing.

How Magnets Heal

(a) All fluids are influenced by the effect of magnets. Ionisation is a process in which molecules are charged (both positively and negatively).

(b) Many physical and chemical properties of water change when exposed to the influence of weak magnetic fields. The changed properties continue to exist for a long time. Namely they are temperature, density and viscosity.

(c) Since blood is also a fluid, it is similarly influenced by the use of magnets and its properties undergo a change.

(d) When fluid containing salts comes in contact with magnetic flux, the physical properties of fluid change. Blood is a fluid matter and many organic salts form its important constituents. The properties of blood change under the influence of magnets. The changed blood coursing through the whole body exerts a beneficial influence on the entire body which helps the body revive and prevent many ailments. Thus, magnets promote health and provide energy by eliminating disorders in the various systems working in the body, stimulating blood circulation and building new cells to rejuvenate the tissues of the body.

Magnetic flux greatly affects magnetic substances like iron and oxygen, with the result that haemoglobin in the blood vessels moves to activate circulation. Magnets help increase the number of new RBCs. The ratio between the RBCs and WBCs is not disturbed but inactive and decayed blood corpuscles are removed and fresh vital blood is pumped into the system.

(e) Magnets promote better breathing action which results in cure and prevention of diseases connected with the circulatory system like bronchitis and asthma.

(f) The internal secretion of hormones is greatly improved by the joint effect of the internal heat of the body and the external heat caused by the magnets. The transmission of blood is facilitated by this heat and also in the capillary vessels which are spread like a net around hormone secretion tubes. The secretion tubes get properly warm and their functions become active by supply of excess oxygen. All diseases caused by lack of hormone secretion are favourably affected and improved by regular and constant use of magnets.

(g) The effect of magnets on the Pituitary gland helps in determining the height of an individual. When there is more secretion, height increases more than usual while less secretion results in height remaining less than normal. Magnets are extremely helpful in increasing the height of boys and girls to some extent up to the age of 14 – 15 years.

(h) Magnets exert a favourable influence on re-formation, resuscitation and promotion of cell growth. The magnetic flux generates a comfortable warm feeling in the body. Consequently remarkable curative effects are noticed in problems like chapped skin, chilblains and incised wounds.

(i) Exert profound influence on diseases like high blood pressure, hardening of arteries, gouty deposits, arthritis, aches and pains.

(j) Strengthen the immunological system through regulation of sodium and potassium in the body.

Types of Magnets Generally Used for Healing

(a) **Strong Healing Magnets**: Power 2000 gauss

(b) **Medium Healing Magnets**: Power of 500 gauss (for use of children or disease like earache, toothache.

(c) **Curved low power Ceramic Magnets**: Power of 200 gauss. For general use above the neck.

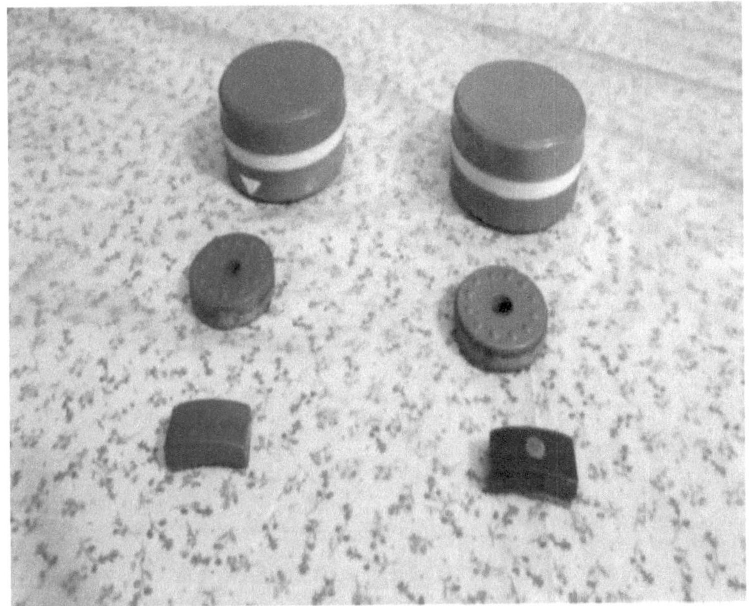

Five Standard Methods of Magnetic Treatment

Method 1

North Pole (Red) under the palm of the right hand and South Pole (Blue) under the palm of the left hand.

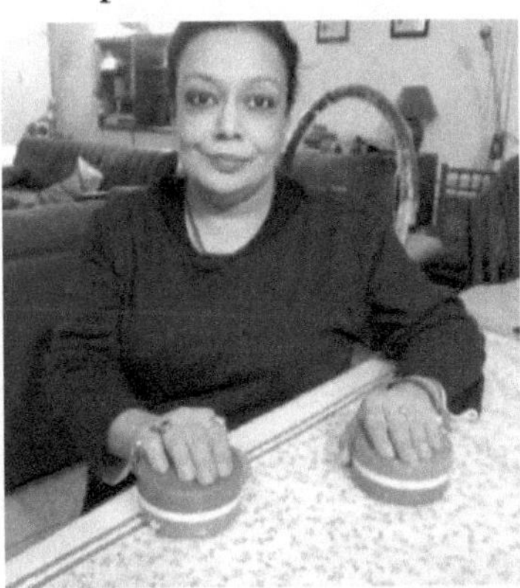

Used for treating ailments of the upper half of the body.

Method II

North Pole (Red) under the palm of the right hand and South Pole (Blue) under the sole of the left foot.

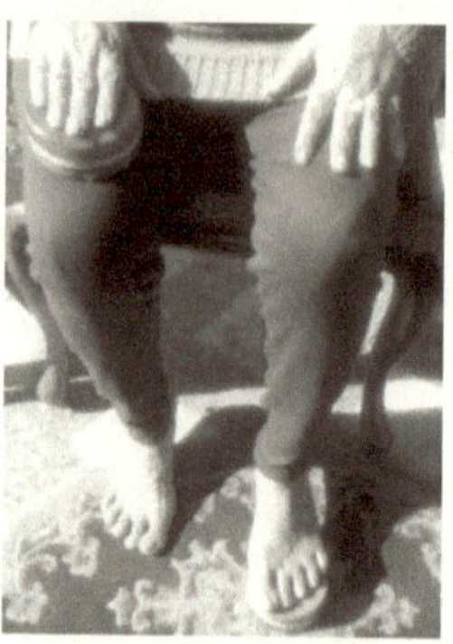

Used for treating ailments of liver, spleen, stomach and intestines. Has a curative effect on the digestive system and cures gastric and other abdominal ailments.

Method III

North Pole (Red) under the palm of the left hand and South Pole (Blue) under the sole of the left foot.

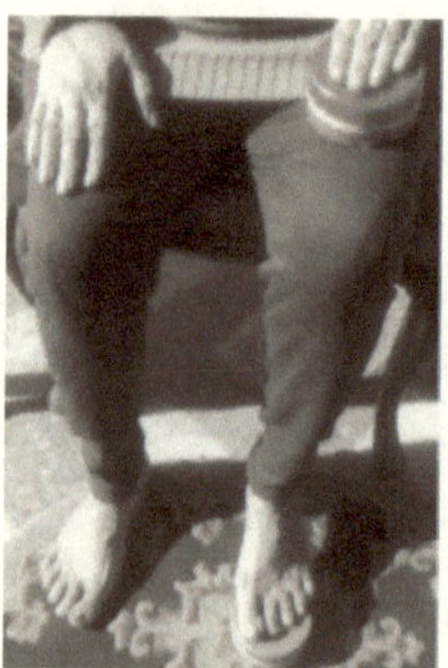

Used for treating left side ailments like paralysis, polio, pain in the left side, general weakness etc.

Method IV

North Pole (Red) under the palm of the right hand and South Pole (Blue) under the pole of the right foot.

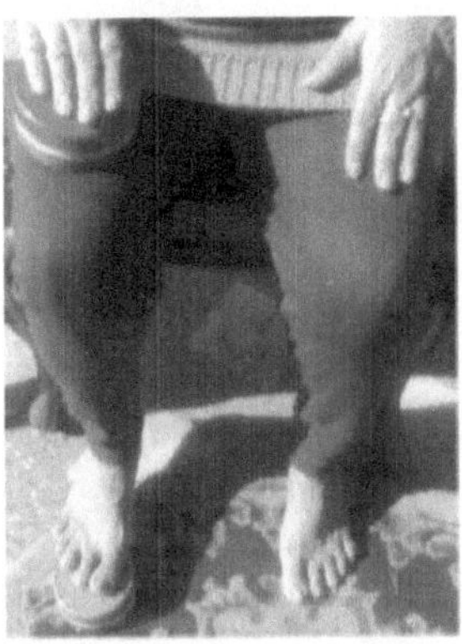

Used for treating ailments on the right side of the body like paralysis, polio, pain in the right side, general weakness etc.

Method V

North Pole (Red) under the sole of the right foot and South Pole (Blue) under the sole of the left foot.

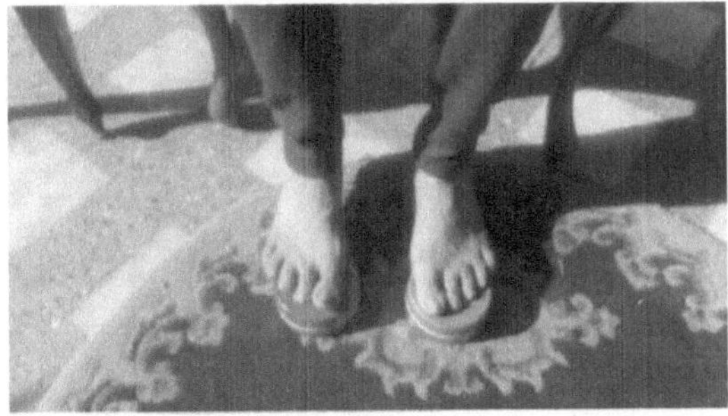

Useful for ailments of the lower parts of the body, including arthritis of feet and ankles, gout, low circulation of blood in the legs.

Basic rule for Application of Magnets:

(a) North Pole is applied on the right side and South Pole is applied on the left side.

(b) When magnets are used in vertical position north is always applied on TOP and south is applied below.

Application of Single Magnet

Many physicians and scientist advocate use of one single pole at a time.

North Pole (Red) may be used alone for:

(a) Arthritis (calcification of joints is slowly dissolved by North Pole).

(b) Bleeding or haemorrhage.

(c) Bleeding of wounds, cuts, bruises.

(d) Broken bones, broken joints, fractures (South pole on the upper and north pole on the lower portion ensures best healing).

(e) High blood pressure (North Pole under the right ear down to the artery).

(f) Infection, pus, discharge (North Pole arrests and nature heals.

(g) Kidney infection or stone.

(h) Sprain in ankles, back, hips, legs and feet.

(i) Teeth and gums (decaying teeth, infection of gums, swelling, pus).

(j) Tooth ache with bad smell, bleeding and wounds.

(k) Biting of bees, insects (North Pole on the affected part).

South Pole may be used for:

(a) All kinds of pain, stiffness in limbs, arms, legs, shoulders, hips etc.

(b) Poor digestion, gas formation.

(c) Less production of insulin (diabetes).

(d) Enlargement of prostate.

(e) Weak muscles.

(f) Hair colouring.

Use of Ceramic Crescent Shaped Magnets

These low power magnets are used on areas above the neck. Normally they are never applied for more than ten minutes at a time. Application can be repeated after a gap of six to eight hours. The points of application are:

(a) For sinusitis, rhinitis—place magnets on either side of the nose (red touching the right side of the nose and blue on the left side).

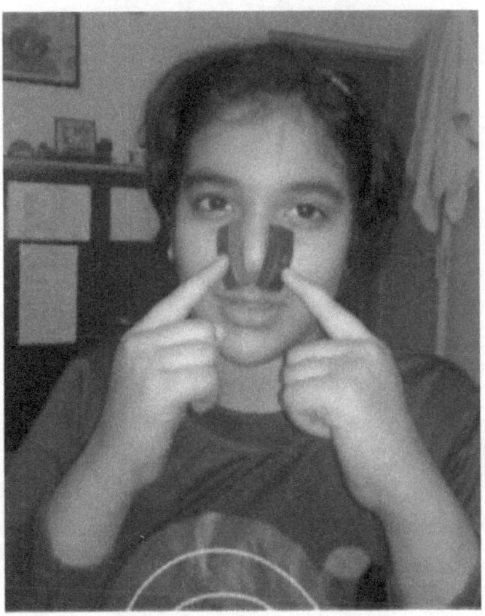

For headaches—place magnets on top of the eyebrows (red on the right side and blue on the left side).

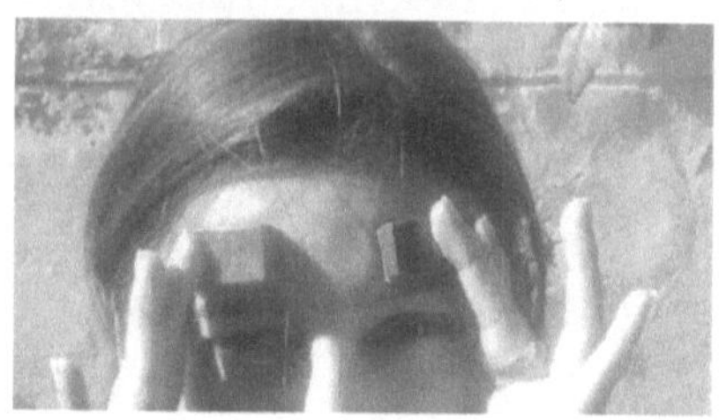

For insomnia—place blue side on the centre of the forehead

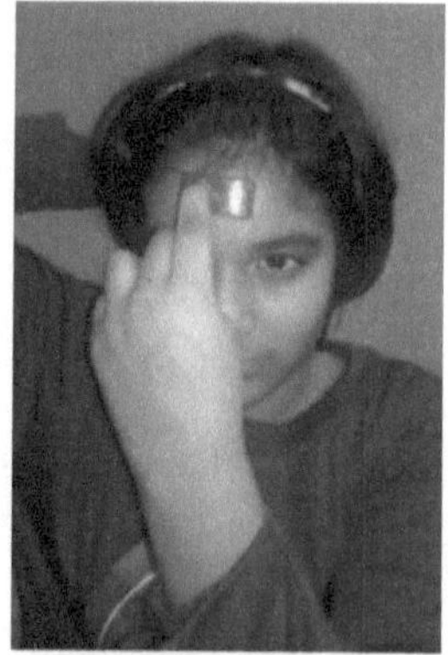

(Red side in front, blue touching forehead)

(b) For ear troubles—place on ear (red on right ear and blue on left ear).

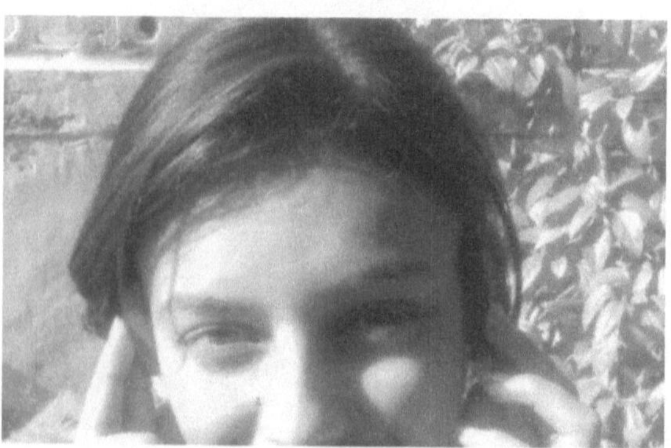

(c) For tonsils—place on throat

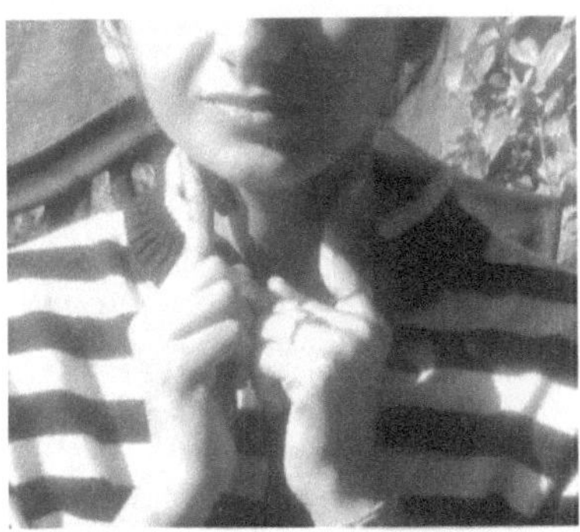

(d) For gaining height in children upto 15 years:

First day—red side on right temple and blue side on left temple (15 mins).

Second day—red side on the frontal forehead and blue side on the back of the head (15 mins).

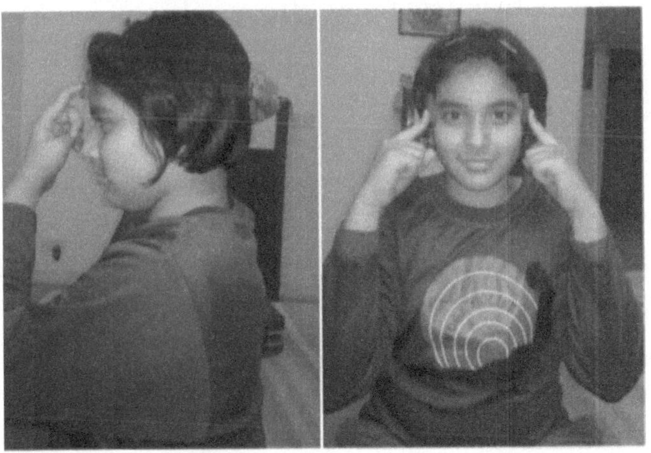

Guidelines and Precautions for use of Magnets

1. Cold Drinks or Cold Food should NOT be taken during or immediately after application of magnets. Wait for **ONE** hour.

2. Avoid cold bath for at least **ONE** hour.

3. Apply magnets **TWO** hours after a regular meal.

4. DO NOT use strong magnets to the region of brain, heart and eyes.

5. Duration of use of ceramic magnets to the head is NOT to exceed TEN minutes.

6. Avoid bringing sophisticated electrical or electronic equipment (TV, mobiles, time pieces) near strong magnets.

7. Ensure fingers are not allowed to come in between when opposite poles of strong magnets are clapped together.

Healing Water

Healing water is nothing but drinkable water treated with magnets. This water is prepared by using the North Pole of a magnet (Red) or the South Pole of a magnet (blue) or by mixing the waters of both in equal quantities.

The water is bestowed with tremendous curative powers and plays an important role in treatment of a large number of ailments. Its effectiveness is unquestionable. Unfortunately its usefulness is not advertised as done for many drinking water appliances.

It is easy to prepare the healing water at home and use it as required.

Healing water made by mixing water treated by both Poles helps to cure the following troubles:

(a) Abscesses and boils

(b) Anaemia (drink thrice daily)

(c) Arthritis

(d) Backache.

(e) Blood Pressure

(f) Colitis (thrice daily)

(g) Conjunctivitis

(h) Constipation

(i) Diabetes

(j) Diarrhoea (25 ml every three hours)

(k) Dyspepsia (thrice daily)

(l) Dysuria (50 ml for times daily)

(m) Eczema

(n) Epilepsy

(o) Fistula

(p) Flatulence

(q) Gall stones(four times daily)

(r) Goitre

(s) Headaches

(t) Height gain

(u) Hepatitis

(v) Hydrocele

(w) Hyperacidity

(x) Insomnia

(y) Jaundice

(z) Kidney stones

(aa) Leucorrhoea

(bb) Malaria (four times in fever, thrice thereafter)

(cc) Menorrhagia

For the following specific ailments, water treated with a single Pole is more beneficial:

South Pole	**North Pole**
Acidity	Colds
Asthma	Constipation
Dysentery	Cataract

Leucorrhoea	Diabetes
Nausea, Vomiting	Dandruff
Prostate	Headaches
Stone	Heart problems
Eye problems	Low blood pressure
Eczema, Skin problems	Nephritis
Gums swelling, bleeding	Measles
High blood pressure	Paralysis
Vertigo	Rheumatism
Insect bites	Sleeplessness
Liver problems	General Energy Booster
Mumps	
General Infection Controller	

Preparation of Magnetized Water

- Take a pair of encased high power magnets of flat surface (3-4").
- Take two glass bottles or jars of clean water.
- Place one on North Pole (red) and other on South Pole (blue).
- Cover the bottles/jars and leave overnight.
- Water gets magnetized in 12 hours.
- Transfer magnetized water to a third container (if mixed water is to be used).
- Use North Pole water/South Pole water separately, if required.

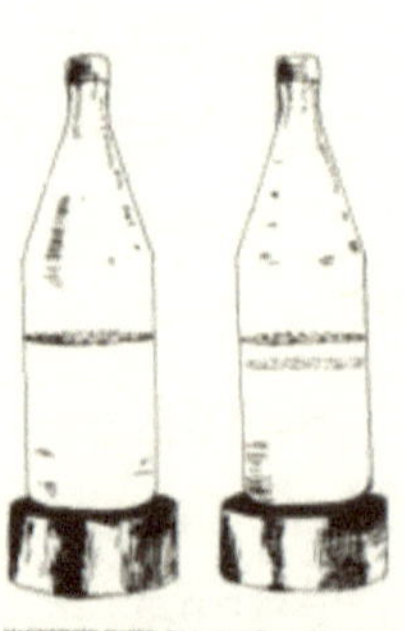

Dosage of Magnetized Water

- Adults – 50ml (2 ounces) at a time. Three times a day. Best taken in the morning, before breakfast and after lunch/dinner.
- Children – (1 ounce) 25 ml thrice daily.
- For ailments – as prescribed.

Note: Do not take in excessive quantity.

CHAPTER 5

Basic Laws of Nature

KEY TO GOOD HEALTH

Breathing

Breathing is an essential part of all human beings. It is the process by which air is taken in. One cannot live without air for more than 4 minutes. Since we need to make no effort to breathe it is taken for granted and its value to the human being at the physical, mental and emotional level is not fully understood. The earlier we appreciate its importance and start to control the rate of breathing the better we will be able to exercise control over one's Self.

It is of immense help in nutrition. To get the maximum value from the foods that we eat air is perhaps the most essential element. Without oxygen that is in the air food will not energize our body. Oxygen combines with Hydrogen and Carbon furnished by the food, the reaction within the body generates heat and provide energy for physical work. Helps in digestion, growth and brain function. While breathing out Co_2 is expelled from the body. Research has shown that the average full breathing rate is 16-18 per minute. Various activities cause the breathing rate to increase.

The best way to maintain good health is to breathe slow and deep. A full inhalation and exhalation will expand and contract the lungs. The two opposite motions make for a balanced breathing system. Breathing helps in the following activities:

A. Balance of autonomic nervous system, which in general terms affects our internal organs.

B. Affects quality of blood through digestion and assimilation.

C. Abdominal breathing and exhalation are connected with blood circulation.

D. Remember when breathing is calm the mind is also at ease.

E. Inhalation expands the lungs, creating a degree of tension.

F. Exhalation contracts the lungs, relaxing nervous activity and loosening the tense body.

G. Holding breath makes for mental concentration.

H. When tense the exhalations are longer and stronger than inhalation.

I. Breathing practice can be undertaken at any time without affecting one's routine.

J. To attain better control of self it is necessary to become conscious of the body process of breathing.

Various methods to control breathing are enunciated by various spiritual gurus. You can practice any of the following as per your convenience:

A. Breathe in and out in the same frame of time i.e. count of four or five.

B. Breathe in and out and give some gap after taking the breath in and after exhalation. Breathe in for 5 seconds, hold for 5 seconds, breathe out in 5 sec., hold breath for 5 sec. Repeat this process 10 times to start with.

C. Take a deep breath in, exhale slowly taking 15 sec. In this exercise the stomach is pulled in to expel all air. Exhalation time can be increased with practice, in order to calm the mind.

D. Practice breathing using the Sudarshan kriya technique:

1. Start with breathing in and out in 5-6 sec. Repeat 20 times.

2. Follow with breathing out more rapidly in 2-3 sec. Repeat 40 times.

3. End with quick exhalation faster than (II) above. Repeat 40 times.

4. The entire process should be repeated thrice.

5. This should be practiced in a calm state of mind at least two to three hours after meals.

Proper Diet

The human body has two main mechanisms. One which nourishes the body and the other which cleanses it by eliminating the remaining refuse through perspiration/sweat, urination, passing of faeces, saliva and tears.

It needs to be emphasised that there are many aspects to a proper diet to achieve the ultimate "HEALTHY YOU".

Before the discussion on other aspects, it is prudent to understand what the body needs, namely:

(a) **Proteins** – for providing building blocks needed for growth, repair and maintenance of the body tissues and organs.

(i) Proteins are composed of more than 70 amino acids.

(ii) For assimilation of food taken, the body releases enzymes into the intestinal tract. Enzymes break protein into amino acids. Muscles, skin, hormones and enzymes are all made of amino acids. Their need is continuous.

Shortage of proteins leads to weakness and fatigue while excess leads to blood vitiating and clotting starts in intestines.

The requirement of proteins depends on body weight. Every Kg. of body weight needs special attention. Proteins found in milk, almonds, nuts, coconut, soya beans, eggs and meat are of high quality. Cereals, pulses, peas and seeds also contain essential amino acids.

(b) **Carbohydrates** – They are compounds of Carbon, Hydrogen and Oxygen.

They are needed to provide heat and energy to the body. Starch and Sugar are the most common Carbohydrates. Both are found in green plants. The starch becomes fat and accumulates in the body. Its digestion puts a strain on the liver. Excess intake causes obesity whereas shortage produces restlessness and weakness. The requirement of carbohydrates for an average person (weight around 70 kg.) is 160-240 gms per day.

(c) **Fats** – They are required as concentrated source of energy and provide fatty acids for lubricating various types of operations within the human body. Some nutritionists recommend that not more than 30% of total calories should be derived from fats.

Fats produce twice as much heat as the same weight of carbohydrates in the process of their oxidation. That energy is transformed into muscular work and body heat. It is hard to quantify the requirement of fats by the average human being. Nutritionists recommend 25-35 gms daily.

(d) **Vitamins** – They are chemical substances required in very small quantities by our bodies. They promote certain chemical processes within the body. They help in processing proteins, carbohydrates and fats etc. so that those elements in our food could perform their functions, like creating energy, building and replacing cells and helping in prevention of diseases, thus promoting good health. It is considered prudent to take vitamins found in fruits and vegetables.

Vitamins can be classed as water soluble (Vitamin C and vitamins in the B complex) because they dissolve readily in water and fat soluble (vitamins A, D, E, K and beta carotene) as these dissolve more readily in oil. Vitamin A comes in two forms. As vitamin A it is found in liver, eggs, butter, cod liver oil and fortified dairy products. As beta carotene it is the phytochemical responsible for the colour of carrots, sweet potatoes, red peppers, apricots, mangoes and peaches. It is necessary for maintaining good vision, the growth of bones and glands, the inner lining of the body, cell membranes and healthy functioning of the immune system. Its deficiency can affect how iron is used by the body. It is depleted by alcohol, cortisone and intestinal, kidney or liver diseases.

B Complex vitamins help to maintain a strong immune system. They are involved in energy production (essential for people with low energy levels and fatigue). They support adrenal glands (one of the major glands connected with stress). These have been found to be helpful in treating peripheral neuralgia (pain in a nerve of the arms, legs, shoulders, neck or scalp).

B-I or thiamine (found in whole grains, meat, fish, poultry, legumes, nuts and seeds) is needed for breakdown of food into energy, hence deficiency of it can lead to fatigue, irritability, sleep disturbance and chest pains. Severe deficiency could result in numbness, cal muscle cramps and leg pain. The recommended supplement is 50 mg per day.

B 3 (Niacin) is obtained from meat, poultry, dairy products, tofu, nuts and seeds. Niacin is known to lower cholesterol levels, aids in the reduction of osteoarthritic inflammation and counters the effects of caffeine. Its deficiency could cause anxiety, fatigue, depression and loss of short-term memory. Adequate daily dose is 20 mg per day.

B 5 (pantothenic acid) is required to maintain optimal energy levels, for wound healing and maintaining strong immune system. It is essential to counter stress. Good sources are eggs, milk, fresh vegetables and bran. The body requires 50 mg per day.

B 6 (pyridoxine) is essential for brain functions, the growth of RBCs, functioning of immune system and prevention and treatment of degenerative diseases. Clinical studies show it helps change pain thresholds. Good sources of B 6 are bananas, chicken, fish, eggs, oats, soyabeans, tomatoes, peanuts and walnuts. Adequate daily dose is 75 mg.

B 12 is a crucial nutrient for healthy nervous system (helping in growth and maintenance of melanin sheath) development of RBCs. Its deficiency is linked to paranoia, restlessness, irritability, memory loss, insomnia. It is found only in animal and dairy products. Its deficiencies can cause loss of balance, numbness and weakness of the limbs, irritability and even depression. Both alcohol and sleeping pills lower B12 levels in the body. The recommended supplementary dose is 100 mcg per day.

Folic acid (a type of B complex) helps in division and replacement of RBCs. Its deficiency causes irritability and gastrointestinal upsets. Good sources of folic acid are dark green leafy vegetables, carrots, apricots, beans, chicken, liver and walnuts. The recommended daily dose is 400 mcg.

Vitamin C is an antioxidant, it neutralises free radicals. In the presence of Vitamin C the body can increase its production of lymphocytes (major infection fighters). Good dietary sources are citrus fruits, strawberries, watermelons, honeydew melons, red peppers, broccoli, sprouts and cauliflowers.

Vitamin D is known as the 'sunshine vitamin'. After exposure to sun it helps the body absorb calcium thus helps bone formation. The natural nutritional sources are eggs, butter, cheese and fish oil. This fat soluble vitamin is stored in the body and excess is harmful. A safe supplement dose is 400 IU.

Vitamin E is found in peanut butter, almonds, sunflower seeds and vegetable oil. It is a potent antioxidant. It boosts synthesis of antibodies and encourages reproduction of lymphocytes, key infection fighting cells. Studies show that taking supplemental Vitamin E significantly reduces the risk of heart disease. The recommended supplement is 800 IU a day.

While supplements have their role, the best source of vitamins is fresh, coloured fruits and vegetables.

(e) **Minerals** – Basic minerals and trace elements are found in food. They are essential for health as protective foods. Details about different minerals are placed below:

Calcium is an important nutrient in pain relief (e.g. leg cramps) and is chiefly supplied by milk products. It works synergistically with vitamin D, phosphorous and magnesium. It nourishes and calms the nervous system. It is an important nutrient for preventing bone loss. It is considered beneficial to take this mineral supplement of 1000 mg daily.

Magnesium normalises the heart rhythm, helps build healthy bones, relieves muscle cramps, balances blood sugar, conducts nerve impulses, enhances the immune system and protects the body from stress. Its deficiency leads to depression, confusion and irritability. It is found in nuts, seeds, tofu, oatmeal, whole grain, seafood and leafy greens. The recommended daily dose is 500 mg.

Potassium, found in all fruits, vegetables, nuts, grains and particularly abundant in bananas, helps to maintain the sodium balance in the body. It is critical for maintaining energy levels and its deficiency leads to lethargy and weakness. If the need arises a supplement of 99 mg a day is recommended.

Iron is necessary to make RBCs, which supply the body with oxygen. Its intake has to be monitored as excess may increase the risk of heart disease and feed pathogens that cause gastrointestinal problems. Good food sources are meat products, legumes, dry fruits. A meal that includes food high in iron should also include vitamin C rich foods to facilitate absorption.

Zinc is present in all organs and is vital to the activity of more than 100 enzymes. Stress depletes it and its deficiency makes it hard to keep the blood sugar level or to digest food. Zinc improves the immune response and helps body utilise vitamin A. Good sources of zinc are chicken, oysters and pumpkin seeds. The daily requirement is 30 mg.

Copper boosts the immune system by making sure your T-cells and antibodies are armed and ready. Sources include shellfish, nuts, sesame seed, mushrooms and wholegrain cereals.

Chromium helps control blood sugar levels, elevated triglycerides, cholesterol. It is found in brewers yeast, wheat germ, rye bread and potatoes.

Balanced Food

It is difficult to standardize a balanced diet. The individual's need for various constituents depends upon several factors:

(a) **Age** – More calories are required at the growing stage as the body has to develop to its optimum level. The requirement declines in old age.

(b) **Nature of routine** – an individual of mainly sedentary routine (like a desk job, less movement at workplace) has a lower requirement of calories than an individual engaged in physical work (like farming, construction labour). Active sportspersons who follow a definite fitness routine have to have a diet plan to be able to perform at optimum level. It is best to consult a nutritionist who can guide one to an optimum diet for maintaining good health.

The following laws of nature help in maintaining 'Healthy You'. Bear in mind these cardinal principles:

(a) Eat minimum sugar

(b) Eat minimum salt

(c) Eat minimum oil

Sugar, glucose and fructose are good as they are simple sugars which get easily digested. Maltose is formed in the mouth when an enzyme in the saliva acts upon starch in the food. Maltose is also split up by an enzyme into a simple sugar i.e. glucose. Sucrose or white cane sugar is different. During the production of white sugar all minerals and vitamins present in sugarcane are either lost or removed. White sugar has only calories. Calcium is needed to digest white sugar. This mineral is obtained by the body from bones if is not available in your food in adequate quantity. This can affect your teeth.

Salt – An ordinary person needs less than half a gram of salt per day. That quantity is easily available to the body from even raw vegetables. Excessive use of salt puts a great strain on the kidneys which have to work overtime to throw the excess salt out. The kidneys of a healthy person cannot throw out more than 4-5 grams of salt per day. The remaining salt remains stored within the body as toxic matter which promotes diseases of the heart, arthritis and high blood pressure. Excess salt also increases the water retaining capacity of the body and causes weight to rise.

Oil – Intake of excess fat is the main cause of large numbers of ailments. Usage of more beneficial oils having a large proportion of polyunsaturated and monounsaturated fatty acids like sunflower oil and corn oil is recommended. Considering the availability of eating joints providing a variety of food choices one has to decide whether one wants to 'Eat to Live' or 'LIVE TO EAT'. To maintain a balanced diet consider the priority: Is your health going to control what you eat or the taste of your tongue?

In the Bhagwat Puran it is written that 'A person who has not controlled his sense organ of taste cannot control his other sense organs. One who has controlled his sense organ of taste can be considered as having already controlled his other sense organs as well.'

One cannot strictly follow a routine. However, the excesses and discretions in the food consumed can be compensated in subsequent meals.

There are many considerations one must be aware of while deciding what to eat, when to eat and how to eat. Some of these are enumerated below:

(a) Eating less is good for health. If more food is taken than what is required it is stored within the body as toxic matter.

(b) Various studies emphasise that 80% of major ailments have the stomach as the root cause. An English proverb says "The glutton digs his own grave with his teeth."

(c) Eat when hungry and drink when thirsty. If a routine is followed, the body would require intake of food at regular times in proper quantity. In today's varied working routines the regular time may vary.

(d) Do not eat between meals. Every time you eat the digestive system has to start its operation even when the previous meal may not have been completely digested.

(e) Do not eat while angry or stressed. Give a gap. The connection between organs of digestion and the vagus nerve means that emotional stress or anger can cause upsets in the alimentary system.

(f) Avoid food for one hour after moderate or severe exercise. Let the life force work fully on one thing at a time.

(g) Chew the food well. Good food tastes better the more you chew. Brown rice, for example, becomes sweeter when chewed well. Chewing well is even more important when one is sick. The digestion of complex carbohydrates begins in the mouth. The more you chew the better is your absorption and assimilation. Complete chewing leads to satisfaction after a meal and thus lessens the desire to overeat.

The following points also need consideration:

(a) Preferably eat fruits and vegetables grown in the climate and area where you live.

(b) Minimize eating of animal protein as the high fat content as well as the antibiotics that animals receive could be injurious to health.

(c) Avoid artificial foods as they include flavouring, colouring and preserving agents.

(d) Minimize consumption of alcoholic beverages and avoid tobacco products in all forms.

(e) Avoid soft drinks and artificially sweetened juices.

(f) Learn the process of healthy cooking.

Proper Elimination

The body mechanism which cleanses it by eliminating refuse and toxic matter is a vital aspect of healthy living. We tend to give more emphasis and importance to the intake of food from its nutritional rather than cleansing aspect.

While food is necessary, not everything that we eat is fully utilized. A certain amount has to be eliminated from the body. The body's elimination process takes one of four routes. The four routes are:

(a) Through the lungs which eliminate carbon and other waste matter with the breath.

(b) Through the kidneys which eliminate water, nitrogen and other toxic matter through urine.

(c) Through the intestines which throw out refuse (including toxic matter) with faeces.

(d) Through sweat and perspiration which get rid of toxins.

Elimination through these routes needs to be kept at the optimal efficient level. Normally, we tend to keep the functioning of only the second and third route in mind and feel satisfied with their functional efficiency. We rarely realize the importance of the cleansing of the lungs and of the skin through perspiration.

Since elimination is intimately linked to the intake of the food, proper diet becomes relevant.

Studies undertaken on the subject reveal that constipation (and diarrhoea to a lesser extent) is one of the major causes of poor health. It is the cause of many ailments. As nerves move the bowels, constipation is both a physical and psychological problem. Carrying waste containing toxins for any length of time is a burden on the body. It becomes a major cause of gas formation.

The weakening of the functioning of the stomach and intestine or chilling in the legs and the lumbar region leads to poor digestion. Material left undigested stimulates the mucous membrane of the colon and accelerates peristalsis, with the result that the contents pass rapidly through the tract before the liquid is adequately absorbed and contents reach the rectum in a semi-fluid state. This causes diarrhoea and dehydrates the body. The process of elimination through lungs can be regulated and controlled with the process of proper breathing (discussed in detail in the chapter on Breathing).

The elimination of toxins through sweat and perspiration can be regulated by keeping the secretory nerves and sweat glands in good health by undertaking daily exercises, according to one's capacity.

To overcome the problem of constipation and diarrhoea it is necessary to press the stomach points and the points in the region of the sigmoid colon. Each point is given pressure for three seconds and all points are treated thrice (see diagram of stomach points). Then the receiver lies face down and the points from T12 to Sacrum are pressed for three seconds each and all points are given pressure three times.

Besides, there are many suggestions to avoid constipation. Some are:

(a) Brisk walk in the morning and evening. Walking produces movement that prevents faeces from remaining stuck to the sides of the intestine and elsewhere.

(b) Take a glass of lukewarm water with lemon in the morning.

(c) Take a glass of warm milk at bed time.

(d) Eat some fruits which are known to reduce constipation. They are papaya, figs, pear, custard apple, guava, tomato and sprouts.

(e) Take enough water (about 8-10 glasses a day).

(f) Eat cereals from which bran has not been removed.

Proper Sleep

Sleep is a natural attribute of the body. It is estimated that human beings spend one third of their time sleeping.

Sleep is that period of inactivity where we are generally unresponsive to our environment. Sufficient sleep is more essential to recover from fatigue and tiredness than any therapy or drug. No matter how static one remains while being awake, the organs continue to function and the muscles remain in a state of tension. However, during sound sleep the organs and the cerebral nerves are at rest and the muscles relax. This enables the body to recover from weakness and one gets up fully refreshed. This is possible if one gets sound sleep.

The brain waves (as recorded by EEG—a biometric device) are generally 20 pulsations per second when one is awake. When one goes to sleep the rate of pulsation drops. In sound sleep it drops to 5 per second. In the dreaming period the rate of pulsation increases to 10 pulsations per second.

The fewer the number of pulsations, the more is the rest felt by the system. During sleep both mind and body should be in a resting stage as this is the time when the body's self-healing mechanism functions. During this period new cells are constructed and old ones recycled.

The dreaming period in sleep is not always a sign of good health. It is a working function and not a sign of rest. It is said that it is the body's way of processing either physical or psychological residues.

Since sleep is one of the essentials for a body's physical and psychological wellbeing, it is vital to understand what causes disruption in sleep. Each of the basic factors influences one other. Food is one aspect. It is essential to know what your diet should be. For proper absorption of food it is essential to have an interval of two hours between eating and sleeping. A very old maxim states, "After dinner walk a mile". Exercise of the body is another important aspect. This activity improves blood circulation and more oxygen burns away the toxicity of the blood. The digestive system is strengthened and expulsion of toxins is ensured. Exercise also stretches and extends your muscles and joints and massages your glands, sense organs and other parts of the body.

Nature has given you a life force (prana) which is ever engaged in preventing diseases and preserving your health. This life force is interlinked with stress. When stress exceeds the normal limit, the life force stops moving within the body in the normal fashion. This impedes proper restful sleep. Unfortunately today's work environment has undergone a sea change. There are no fixed hours of work. Higher targets and time limits to achieve them cause stress and tension. As a result work pressure remains in the body and mind even after working hours.

Work schedules also affect sleep. Today's life is a 24x7 phenomenon. A sizeable number of people are working through the night. The body has to be conditioned to adjust its daily routine so that one gets adequate sleep and rest and remains healthy. Body stress is a state of mind. The first act should be to pacify the mind. When you sit for contemplation and meditation both the inhalation of oxygen and the metabolic rate go down and the blood pressure also reduces. There are different techniques to meditate and look within. If practised in a correct manner they are effective. Some of these techniques do not take more than ten minutes and can be practiced even at the workplace. Three such techniques are:

(a) Instant relaxation technique. Time taken 3 to 4 minutes.

(b) Quick relaxation technique. Time taken 3 to 4 minutes.

(c) Deep relaxation technique. Time taken 3 to 4 minutes.

The detailed technique for each is placed below.

Instant relaxation technique

(a) Join heels and toes, arms by side of body

(b) Tighten the toes. Pause two secs. Then tighten the ankle joints.

(c) Stretch calf muscles. Pause two secs.

(d) Pull knee caps. Pause two secs. Then tighten thigh muscles.

(e) Exhale and pull inwards your abdominal muscles.

(f) Form fists and tighten them. Stretch arms.

(g) Inhale and expand face.

(h) Tighten. Pause two secs. Tighten. Pause. Tighten. Pause

(i) Release whole body and relax.

Quick relaxation technique

(a) Lie down on ground or sit in chair allowing back to rest fully. Let whole body collapse, legs apart, arms away from waist, facing upwards.

(b) Observe your abdominal muscles bulging up and sinking down. Movements automatically get regularised and slow. Count ten cycles.

(c) Watch yourself inhale and exhale. Inhale, feel the air go deep into the lungs and exhale fully, emptying the lungs. Repeat without forcing the breathing, simply observe and feel the natural breathing process. Count ten cycles.

(d) Feel the following effects: observe the body collapse as you exhale and the abdominal muscles go down, then come up. Feel body becoming light and energetic as you inhale fully. The body relaxes while inhaling and feels energised while exhaling. Repeat for ten cycles.

Deep relaxation technique

(a) Lie supine on ground or relax in a chair. Watch the body relax from toes to head. Observing yourself relax the body part by part induces deep and full relaxation.

These three relaxation techniques are powerful ways of coping with stress and controlling tension related problems like high blood pressure and insomnia.

Some of the other techniques to induce sleep are enumerated here. Not all may be applicable to everyone. Select some and practice to benefit.

(a) Sleep is an action of the nerves and an attribute of the mind. While lying in bed bring both hands close to each other. Join the tips of the fingers of both hands. Press together for 10 - 15 seconds.

(b) Press the web between the thumb and the first finger of both hands for 10 -15 seconds. This could be repeated two to three times daily.

(c) Place your fingers behind the ear between the jaw bone and the lower portion of the skull bone ending behind the ear. Press the carotid sinus straight down for 2 -3 cms at least five times.

(d) Place small ceramic (ENT) magnets over the eyebrows for 15 minutes, close your eyes and breathe in and out in even time (breathe in to a count of four and breathe out in the same time). Let the breathing be normal and not forced.

(e) Place blue ceramic magnet in the centre of the forehead for about 10 minutes while preparing to go to sleep.

(f) Another recommended technique is to lie down, relax the body and start breathing slowly and steadily. Now count slowly from 100 backwards.

Select and practise techniques which suit you and enable you to get proper sleep.

Exercise

The human body is designed to sustain itself. Exercise is most necessary for the body to maintain, repair and improve itself.

To understand the necessity of exercise ponder over the following:

(a) Movement of the body helps take in more air and oxygen into the system so that various parts of the body can draw strength from it.

(b) It strengthens the bones, slows down the progress of osteoporosis, strengthens and tones the muscles.

(c) It imparts flexibility to joints, tendons and ligaments.

(d) It massages your glands, sense organs and other vital parts of the body (Spine for example).

(e) It improves blood circulation and makes oxygen burn away the toxicity of the blood.

(f) Helps to strengthen the digestive system and ensures expulsion of toxins. Today lifestyles are governed by automation. Many activities for which one had to exert and move the body no longer require physical labour. For example people today prefer to use vehicles for movement even for a short distance. Earlier, in households most of the cooking was done sitting on the floor. The person had to sit and get up a number of times while cooking each meal. Today cooking is done standing up. Eating also required sitting on the floor but today we sit on chairs and movement is minimal. Sitting on the floor enabled movement of the leg joints and lower back and exercised the joints, ligaments and spine.

Our oxygen intake is somewhat related to our pulse rate. Pulse rate goes up with exercise. It is however desirable to keep the pulse rate within certain permissible limits (which vary as per age) while exercising.

	Age	Minimum required pulse rate	Maximum permissible pulse rate
A	Upto 20 Years	100	150
B	Upto 30 Years	100	140
C	Upto 40 Years	100	135
D	Upto 50 Years	95	130
E	Upto 60 Years	95	130
F	Upto 70 Years	85	110
G	Above 70 Years	80	105

Average pulse rate in the above age groups is 70 – 80 per minute. While undertaking any exercise the target is to reach the minimum permissible limit and then maintain it below the maximum permissible limit. The exercise can vary from walking, jogging, running, cycling, rope skipping to outdoor sports. Should it not be possible to undertake any of the above mentioned activities, one variation could be to climb 10 steps of a staircase and come down at the same pace as going up. Keep repeating this exercise till you feel out of breath. This exercises the lower limbs and abdomen.

Similarly, the upper body and upper arms need to be exercised to keep them in shape. Keeping muscles, joints and ligaments in good shape will enable you to perform you daily chores without any problem.

Amongst the many outdoor exercises swimming, cycling, running, jogging may be undertaken as per choice. To maintain good health especially amongst women it is essential to undertake activities where squatting or sitting on the floor and getting up are involved. Joint stiffness, menstruation problems and the tendency to put on weight around the waist and hips is taken care of.

Good Sex

It is observed in nature that all creatures indulge in the sexual union to reproduce and ensure the continuation of the species.

The other function of sex is pleasure. Intimacy with another makes one happy and helps build relationship, understanding and commitment. It paves the way for good communication. Good sex is a two-way act where both partners commit and participate to not only derive personal pleasure but also ensure satisfaction by the other. It lays the foundation for physical, mental and emotional stability.

However, the basics get flouted quite often leading to relationship discord. Problems arise where individuals make personal pleasure of sexual intercourse their only goal at the expense of commitment, understanding, love and intimacy.

Then there are cases of single individuals including juveniles whose bodily problems make them ever ready for sexual contact at every available opportunity. This leads to gang rapes and other sexual crimes.

Lack of harmony becomes the root cause of separations and divorces leading to resentments and frustrations in individuals.

To sum up, the root cause of all sexual problems could be any of the following:

(a) Lack of proper communication and sexual incompatibility between the couple.

(b) Lack of proper education about sex, as this is still not an openly talked about subject.

(c) Disharmonious functioning of some of the endocrine glands (see chapter on endocrine glands).

The solution may lie in:

(a) Imparting education about sex in schools.

(b) Families and close relatives and friends ensuring that harmonious relations exist between the couple.

(c) Harsh and speedy punishments for sexual crimes even for juveniles.

(d) Ensure daily pressing of the seven endocrine glands to restore balance amongst them. This is essential for teenagers with mood swings. In girls it will stimulate regular and proper menstruation, thereby ensuring proper growth and development of the body.

Self Awareness

Our will, the sense of direction and happiness are the totality of the functions of the body, mind and spirit (emotions). It is the holistic approach that made WHO define total health as the stability and balance of body, mind and emotions.

We are all aware that there is a flow of energy in the body as long as we are alive. This energy or 'prana' flows through the channels from toes and fingertips to the top of the head. It is passing through the entire body through a network covering all the organs and the different systems in the body. However control of the body functions and thought rest with the brain which serves as the central controller. The brain is the uppermost and most YIN part of the body.

The brain controls all body functions. In the same way the condition of any of the body parts affects the brain. The messages from the brain to the body and from the body to the brain are a continuous process. The link between the two lies in the neck area.

Our sense organs (sight, smell, touch, hearing and taste) may be considered as receptors of stimuli from the external environment. They transmit the received messages to the brain through the energy channels within the body. It is because of this connection that the emotions produced in the brain as a response to various stimuli could affect and disturb the function of some parts of the body. For the sake of good health it is very important that due attention is given to keep the neck flexible and relaxed.

According to the ancient oriental thinking various emotions are connected with different organs of the body. For example, anger affects the liver, thinking and pensiveness affects the spleen, joy affects the heart, sorrow is associated with the lungs and fear is associated with the kidneys.

One must control the emotions to remain disease free and healthy. Six of the meridians have their start/end points on the face. A couple of minutes spent every day to press these points would indicate what action to take to restore balance in the system and avoid any ailment. The physical brain influences thinking and judgement. If our thinking has to be clear and accurate, we have to rely on our brain.

While we think big on issues related to the external environment, it is prudent to be aware of the brain as related to SELF so that taking due precautions we retain our balance and calm while tackling problems.

CHAPTER 6

Some Points for Preventing Ailments

Having elaborated on all aspects related to health, wellness and fitness, there is a need to emphasise all that one can do to prevent ailments.

Irrespective of your job profile, family background, your surroundings I reiterate that one has to think of SELF a little more often. Take out some time and do some of the activities mentioned below. Not all people remain healthy at all times, due to various factors, they tend to incur some diseases.

Thinking about SELF may involve in some changes in the lifestyle. If your health is your paramount concern you would give a serious thought to the points given below and include some of them in your daily routine.

Key Points for maintenance of health:

1. The endocrine glands in balance help in mental, physical and emotional stability. The seven points either on hand or foot need pressure for 1-2 minutes each.

2. Since major points of the body are in the palms and soles of the feet, it does not take long to press them. Clap your hands at least ten times at a time daily. This activity can be repeated often.

3. Lie down on the back keeping the arms straight by the sides. The legs must be straight and toes pointing upwards. The

two big toes must be level. If they are not it indicates some disturbance in the solar plexus. If the centre shifts upwards one could be suffering from gas formation and constipation and the downward shift leads to frequent motions.

Rectification of solar plexus imbalance:

(a) Lie down on your back with legs straight and arms by your side, toes pointing upwards. Ask someone to apply pressure on the knees. Another person can hold the two big toes and try to pull them up so that the two toes become level.

(b) Sit on the ground or any hard surface with back straight and legs stretched out. Bend one leg and place it over the other just above the knee. Hold the foot with one hand and press the bent leg downwards with the other three to four times. Repeat with the other leg. The displacement of the umbilicus would be rectified.

(c) Sit straight. Stretch out one arm parallel to the shoulder. Place the side of the hand (little finger side) on the elbow of the outstretched hand. Bend the stretched arm and try to touch the thumb with the shoulder edge with a jerk. Repeat this three to four times. Now repeat the exercise with the other arm. This should help rectify the fault.

CHAPTER 7

Healing on Your Fingertips

Like all things in the world our body is made up of five elements. Fingers represent these elements as given below:

(a) Thumb – Fire (Agni)

(b) Index finger – Air (Vayu)

(c) Middle finger – Sky (Shunya)

(d) Ring finger – Earth (Prithvi)

(e) Little finger – Water (Jal)

Health depends upon balance of the five elements. Any imbalance leading to ailment can be removed and cured effectively through the following methods:

Dhyan mudra – put the tips of index finger and thumb together. Keep the remaining three fingers straight. Time 30 minutes.

Benefits: (a) ailments connected with brain (b) sleeplessness (c) loss of memory (d) lack of concentration.

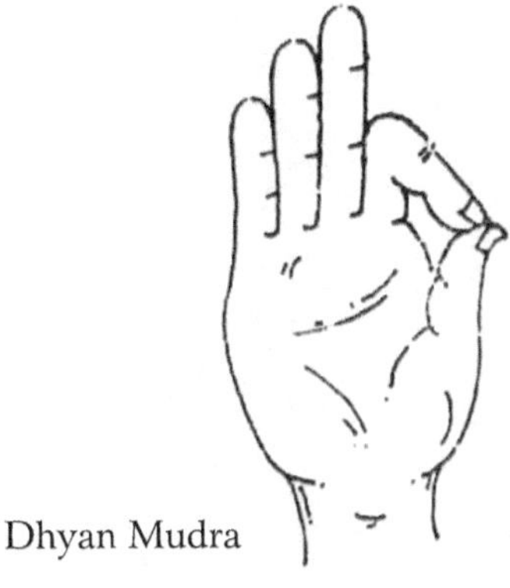

Dhyan Mudra

Prithvi mudra – put tips of ring finger and thumb together. Keep the remaining three fingers straight. Time 30 minutes

Benefits: (a) cures weakness of mind and body (b) gives peace of mind (c) injects chetna in body (d) gives new life to an ailing person

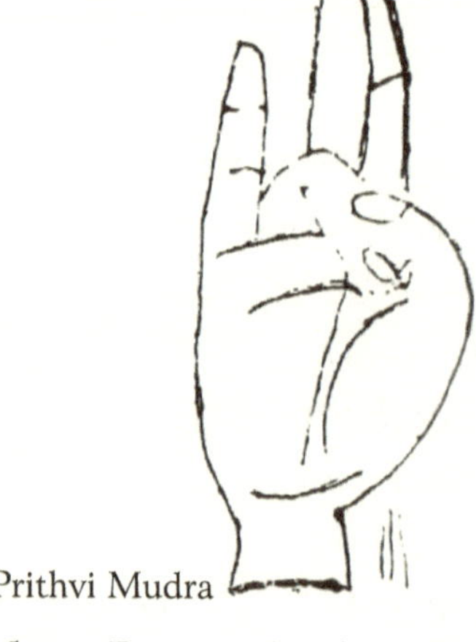

Prithvi Mudra

Vayu mudra – Press index fingertip on base of thumb and keep thumb on finger. Keep the remaining three fingers straight. Time 30 minutes

Benefits: Helps cure (a) rheumatism (b) arthritis (c) gout (d) paralysis (e) Parkinsons disease (f) blood circulatory defects

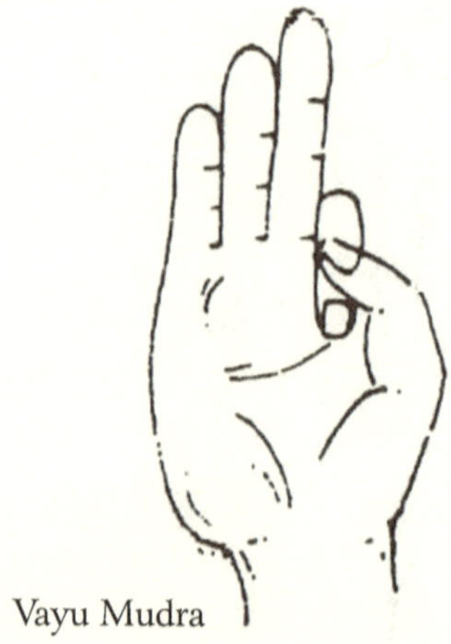

Vayu Mudra

Shunya mudra – Put middle fingertip on base of thumb and put thumb on finger. Keep the remaining three fingers straight. Time 30 minutes

Benefits: Helps cure (a) earache (b) deafness (c) ear infection

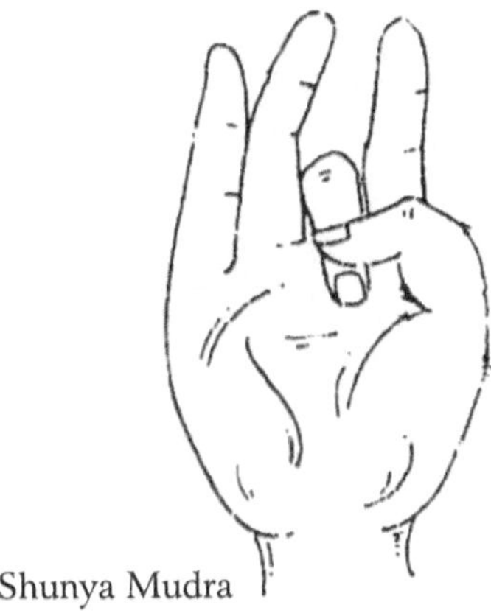

Shunya Mudra

Varun mudra – Join tips of thumb and little finger. Keep the remaining three fingers straight. Time 30 minutes

Benefits: Helps cure diseases connected with shortage of water (b) blood impurities (c) skin diseases (d) acne and pimples.

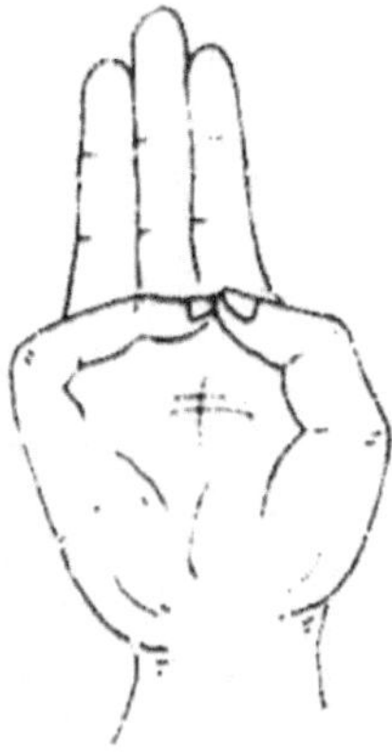

Varun Mudra

Hriday mudra – Put index finger between the point on the edge of the thumb and index finger. Keep tips of middle and ring finger on tip of thumb. Keep little finger straight. Time 30 minutes

Benefits: helps cure (a) heart problems (b) blockage of arteries and valves (c) asthma

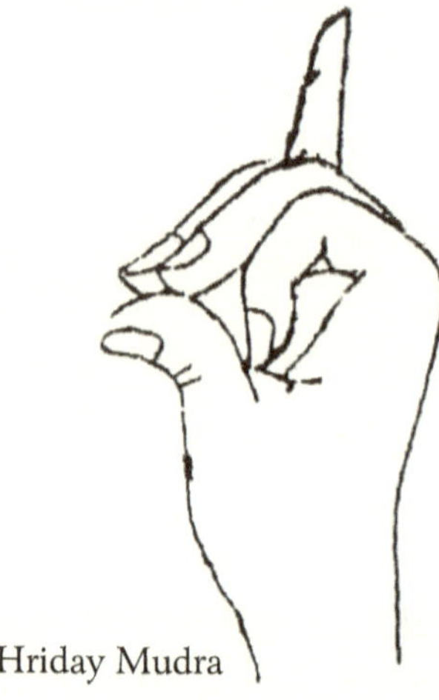

Hriday Mudra

Prana mudra – touch tip of little and ring finger on tip of thumb. Keep the remaining fingers straight. Time 30 minutes

Benefits: helps cure (a) mental weakness (b) physical weakness (c) eye infection (d) brings lustre to eyes, face and body

Prana Mudra

Ling mudra – interlock fingers of both hands together, left thumb encircled by right thumb and index finger. Time 30 minutes

Benefits: helps cure (a) lung congestion (b) cold (c) fever (d) phlegm in chest and lungs

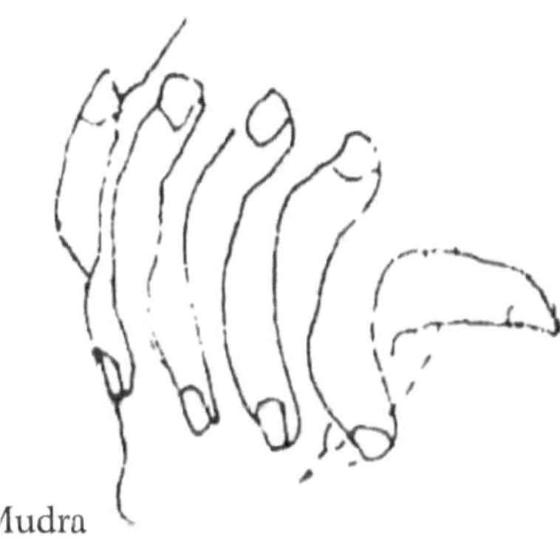

Ling Mudra

Surya mudra – put ring fingertip at base of thumb. Use thumb to press down ring finger. Keep the remaining three fingers straight. Time 30 minutes

Benefits: helps reduce excess fat in body (b) reduces blood cholesterol level

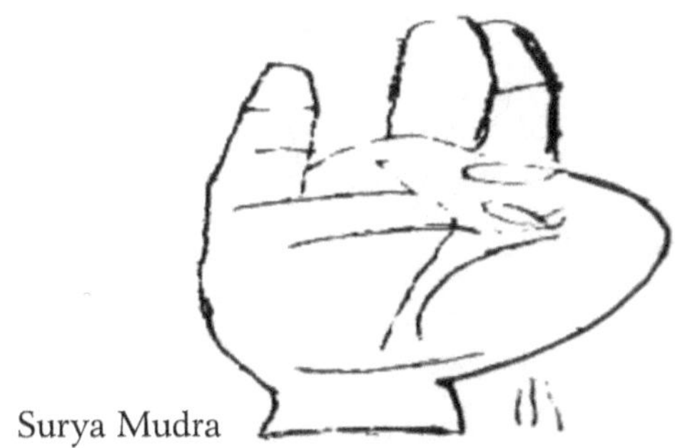

Surya Mudra

Apan mudra – join tips of thumb, middle and ring finger. Keep the remaining fingers straight. Time 30 minutes

Benefits: helps cure (a) constipation (b) indigestion (c) helps free bowel movement

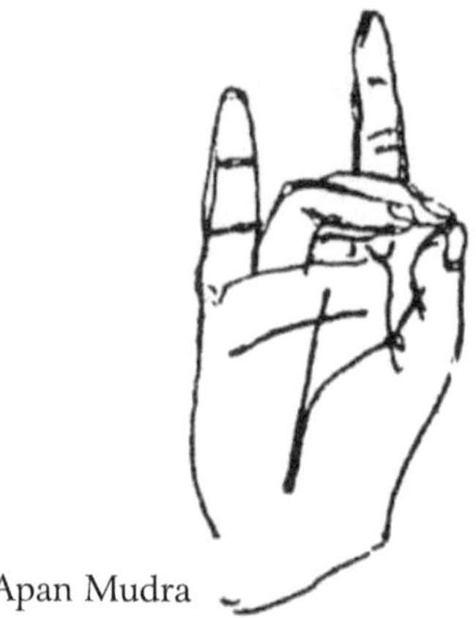

Apan Mudra

Sakat mudra – touch tips of both thumbs together. Keep index finger straight but not joining. Keep other fingers half bent. Time 30 minutes

Benefits: helps to (a) calm the mind (b) curb anger (c) cures hypertension.

Sakat Mudra

CHAPTER 8

Seven Steps Yoga Workout

The benefits of yoga kick in from the moment you calm your mind and inhale deeply.

Trainers demonstrate basic postures (asans) that boost blood circulation, relieve back and neck pain, increase muscle strength, maintain hormonal balance, build immunity and improves mood among others. A word of caution though start supervision if you are over 35 years, have never exercised, or have a medical condition.

1st – SARVANGASANA (The Shoulder-stand)

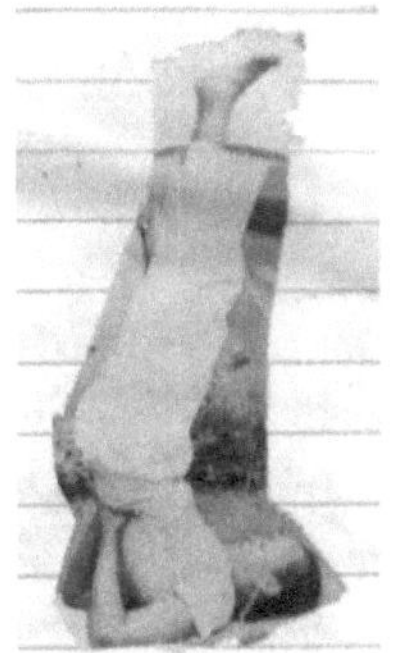

BENEFITS: Stretches the neck and upper-back and strengthen the lower back. Stimulates the thyroid and Parathyroid glands and relieves stress – related tension from neck and shoulders.

WHO SHOULDN'T ATTEMPT: People with CHRONIC HIGH Blood Pressure, menstruating women.

2nd ARDH-MATSYENDRASANA (The HALF SPINAL TWIST)

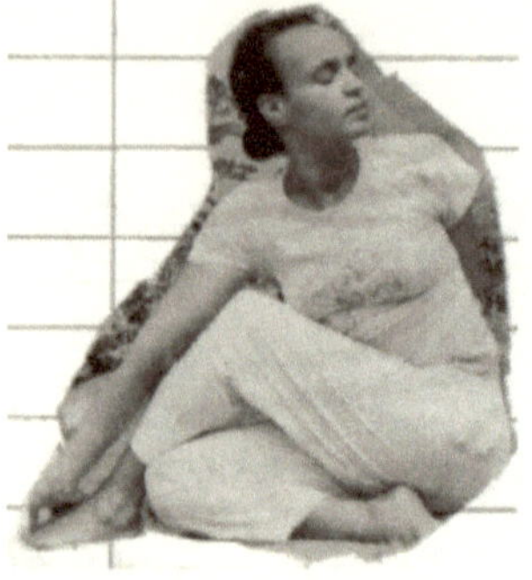

BENEFITS: Combats curvature of the spine, strengthens the hip joint and back muscles and relieves constipation, boosts peripheral nervous system and increase long capacity.

WHO SHOULDN'T ATTEMPT: People with serious spine injury.

3rd HALASANA (The Plough)

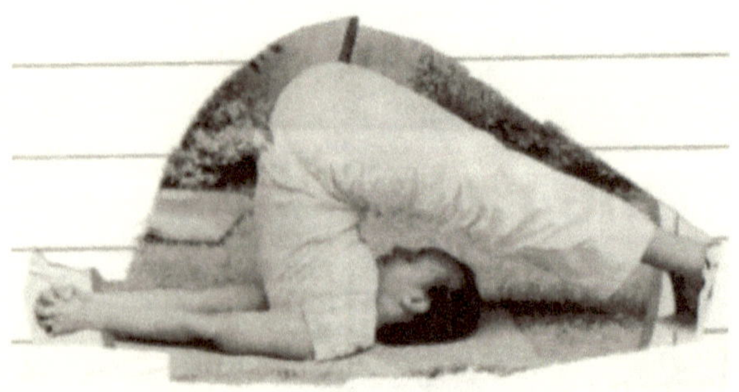

BENEFITS: Corrects posture; massages abdominal organs, relaxes nerves, relieves tension in the neck and back stretches the ligaments and muscles in the calves and thighs.

WHO SHOULDN'T ATTEMPT: Menstruating women.

4th DHANURASANA (THE BOW)

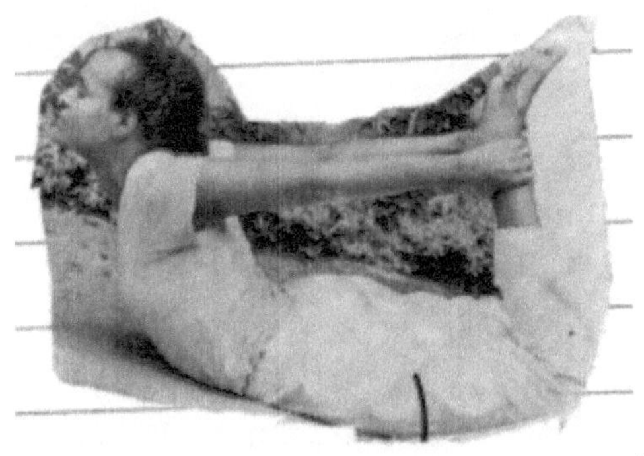

Stretches the thoracic muscles, strengthens the thighs, alleviates stress, stimulates the pancreas to prevent diabetes.

WHO SHOULDN'T ATTEMPT: People with chronic high or low blood pressure, pregnant women.

5th MATSYASANA (THE FISH)

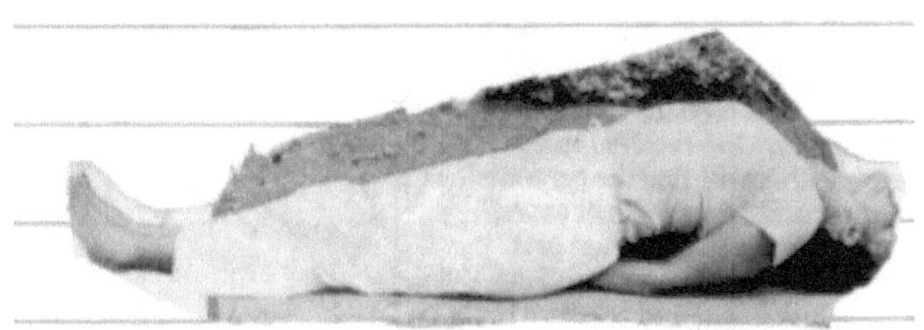

BENEFITS: Strengthens spine and arms, straightens spine curvature, stretches thoracic muscles, improves immunity by gently pressing the thymus gland, and relieves chronic bronchitis and asthma.

WHO SHOULDN'T ATTEMPT: People with serious lower back or neck injury.

6th SALBHASANA (THE LOCUST)

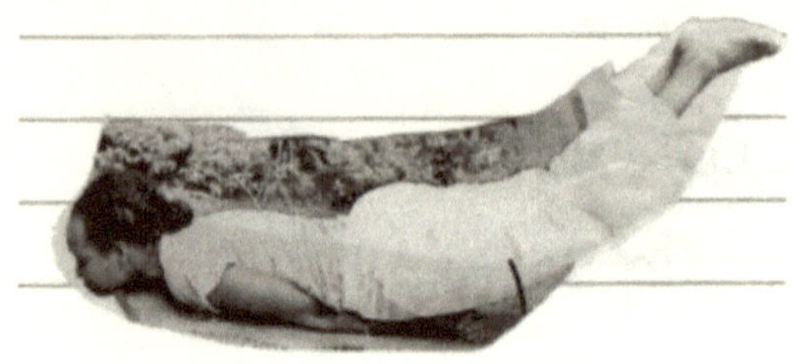

BENEFITS: Builds flexibility and strengthens the back. Also boosts blood circulation and improves digestion.

WHO SHOULDN'T ATTEMPT: People with serious neck or back injury.

7th PASCHIMOTTANASANA (The FORWARD BEND)

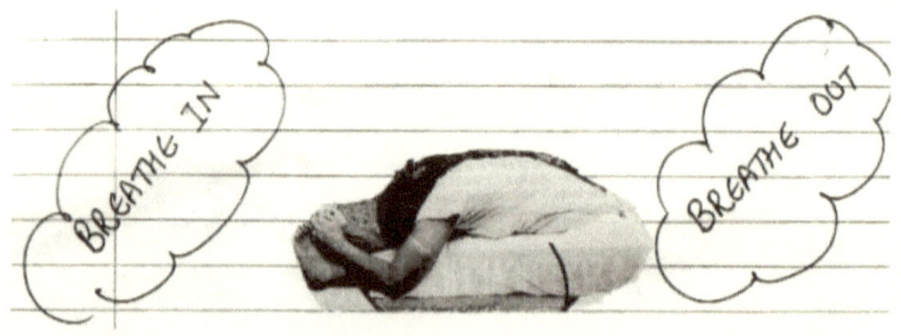

BENEFITS: Strengthen posture, stretches the body from toes to upper back. Prevents Diabetes.

WHO SHOULDN'T ATTEMPT: People with serious lower back injury.

CHAPTER 9

Daily Use of Magnets

Magnets are more than a means of treating ailments and injuries. They should be given the place of treatment plus. This means that they should be used on a daily basis, without disturbing your schedule. I assume that, having read so far, you are by now convinced of the need for self awareness and the powers of magnets and willing to enmesh some of the following suggestions in your daily routine:

My suggestions are:

(a) Use high power magnets under your feet for 15-20 minutes. This can be done while watching TV or even at your workplace if you have a desk job.

(b) Place the small ceramic magnets on your forehead above the eyebrows for ten minutes.

(c) Drink Magnetic Water (50 ml.) three times a day.

(d) Occasionally wash your hair with magnetic water to help it retain colour. There have been cases where grey hair has turned black over a period of time with this treatment.

(e) Wash your face with Magnetic Water whenever convenient.

(f) As you prepare to sleep place high power magnets under your palms for 15-20 minutes.

(g) Place a south pole (blue) magnet under your pillow for a sound sleep.

(h) Those who spend more time in sedentary postures could use a magnetic chair backrest and magnetic cushion on the seat.

CHAPTER 10

Importance of Master Points

There are over a thousand points in our body divided in fourteen meridians that carry the vital force "Prana". Each meridian passes through different parts of the body and has a number of points which relate to the area/organ it touches enroute. Any disturbance in the flow of energy results in imbalance between Yin and Yang. This imbalance causes ailments which is discernable by the pain at one or more points when pressed. The cure is in the repeated pressure on the same points. Thus the diagnosis and the cure lies in the pressure on the relevant points. One could argue that by regular and timed pressure on could avoid ailments but how many points can one press regularly?

There are however a certain number of points which indicate and diagnose more than one, if not many ailments. A summary of the number of ailments each point is effective for is placed below for your perusal. Must we look at the ailments and then press these points? These points need regular pressure to ward of ailments and maintain good health. May you make a habit of pressing these points regularly and reap benefits (keep good health).

There are seven points which are effective in curing a number of ailments each if a regular pressure is given. The seven points known as the Master Points are given here:

The Master Points

1 LU7   One and a half inches above radius stylus process. 2" above volar wrist (thumb side). Useful for treating 15 ailments.

2 LI4   Near the junction of thumb and index finger metacarpal bones. Useful for treating 42 ailments.

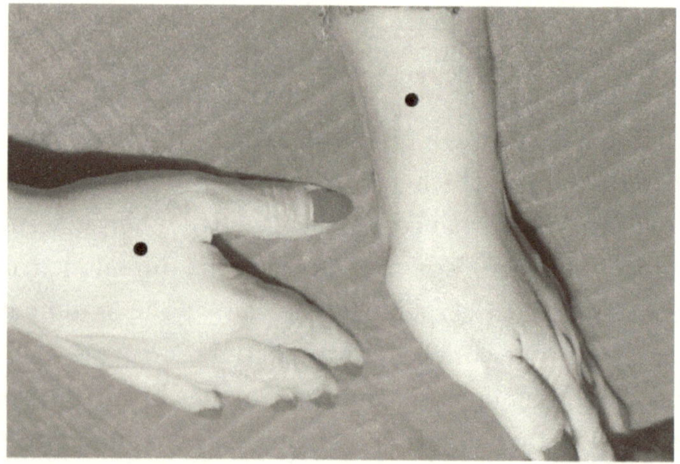

3 GB30   Depression at base of skull between SCM and trapius muscles. Useful for treating 18 ailments.

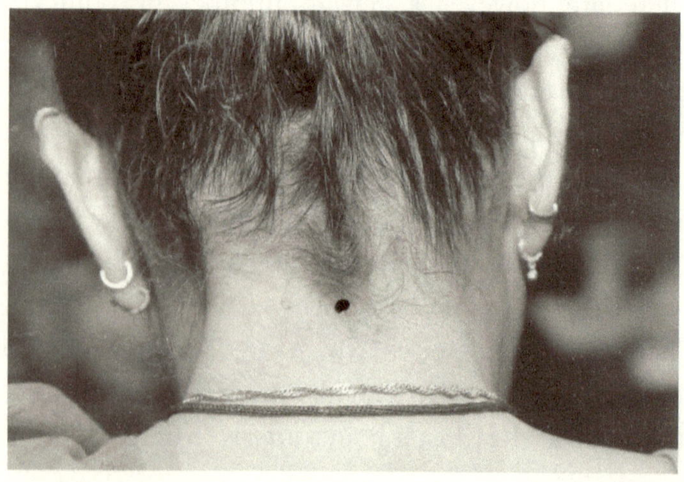

4 St36 On lateral aspect of leg below knee (in a depression) on the anterolateral leg between fibial tuberosity and head of fibula.
Useful for treating 48 ailments.

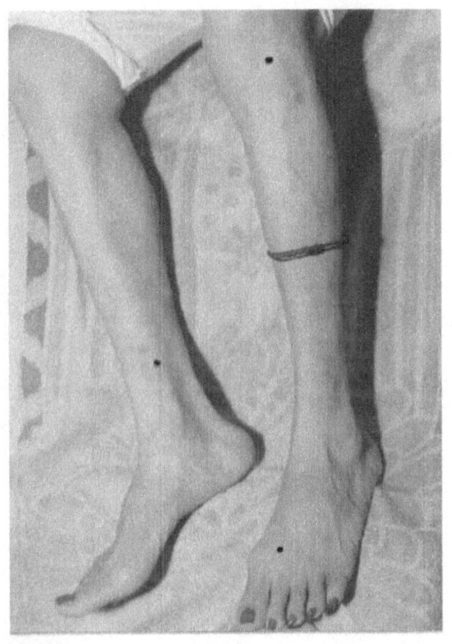

5 BL54 In middle of popliteal fossa on both legs. Useful for treating 11 ailments.

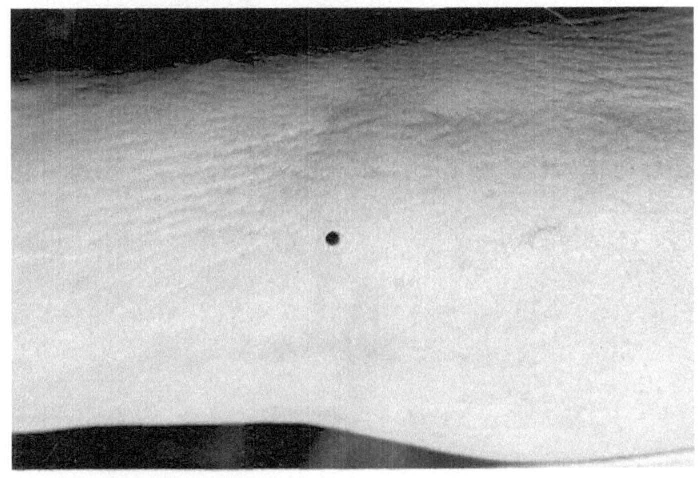

6 Sp6   On inside of leg 3" up from medial malleolus (ankle bone) on posterior border of tibia. Useful for treating 11 ailments.

7 LV3   Two inches above web between first and second toe. Useful for treating 39 ailments.

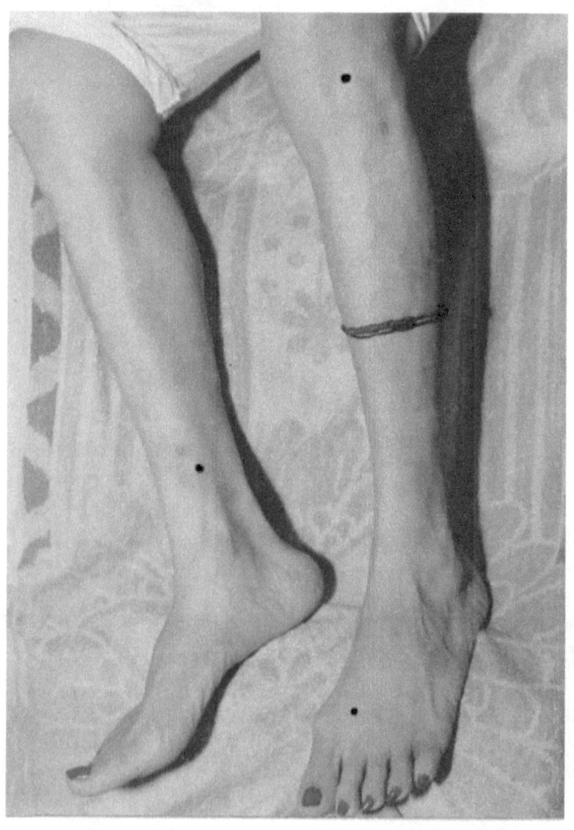

AILMENTS and MASTER POINTS

ASTHMA – 1, 7
ALLERGIES – 2,7
APHASIA – 2
ARTERIOSCLEROSIS – 2, 4
ALZHEIMERS – 3
ANEMIA – 4
ABDOMINAL PAIN – 4
ALCOHOLISM – 4
ANXIETY – 7
ARTHRITIS – 2

BELLS PALSY – 2, 4
BODY SEDATION – 2
BREAST ENLARGEMENT – 4
BRONCHITIS – 1

CATARACT – 2
CERVICAL SPASM – 2
CHOLECYSTIS – 3
COMMON COLD – 1,2,3
CONSTIPATION – 7
COUGH – 1

DEAFNESS – 2,3
DEPUYTRIN CONTRACTURE – 1,4,6,7
DERMATOLOGIC CONDITION – 2,5
 DETOXIFICATION – 7
DIZZINESS – 2, 7
DIVERITICULITIS – 2,4
DIARRHOEA – 4,5
DIGESTION – 4
DYSMENORRHEA – 4
DRUG ABUSE – 7
DIABETES – 4,7
DYSURIA – 6

ENURESIS – 1
EMPHYSEMA – 1,7
EYE DISEASE – 2
EDEMA – 4,6
EPILEPSY – 7

FACIAL PALSY – 2
FEMALE STERILITY—6
FLU –2
FEVER –2

GASTRITIS – 4
GOUT –2,4
GASTROINTESTINAL
GENERAL MUSCLE TONE –4
GALL BLADDER DISEASE –4

HEADACHES – 1,2,3,5
HYPOGLYCEMIA – 2,4,7
HYPERTENSION – 2,3,4,5
HIVES – 4
HEPATITIS – 4,7
HIP PAIN – 5
HOT FLUSHES –6

IMPOTENCY – 4,6
INTERMITTENT CLAODICATION – 5,7
INCONTINENCE – 6
INDIGESTION –2
INSOMNIA – 4,7
ILEOCECAL VALVE – 1,2
INFECTIONS –
IMMUNE SYSTEMS –2,4

JAUNDICE – 4,7

KNEE PAIN – 4,5,7

LEG PAIN – 5
LEUKEMIA – 4,7
LUPUS – 7

MENOPAUSE – 2,5
MENSTRUAL PROBLEMS – 7
MEDIAN NERVE PARALYSIS – 2,4
MIGRAINE – 2,3,7
MULITPLE SCLEROSIS – 3,4
MORNING SICKNESS – 4,7
MORTONS NEUROMA – 7
MUMPS – 2

NEPHRITIS – 4
NERVOUSNESS – 2,3,4
NEURASTHANIA – 2,3,7
NECK PAIN – 1,3,4
NAUSEA – 1,4

PHARYNGITIS – 2
PROSTATITIS – 4
PARKINSONS – 2,3,4,7
PROBLEM—2
PLEURISY TORTICELLIS – 1,4

RHINITIS – 3,5
REPRODUCTIVE DISEASES – 3,5

STERILITY (FEMALE) – 2,7
SMOKING ADDICTION – 1,2,47
STRESS – 2
SCIATICA – 5,6
SINUSITIS – 1,2,3
STOMATITIS – 3

TINNITUS –2,3,7
TREMORS – 4,7
THYROID DISEASE – 1,4,7
TONISILITIS – 3,4
TRIGEMINAL NEURALGIA – 1,2

ULCERS – 4
URTICARIA – 4

VARICOSE VEINS – 6,7
VAGINITIS – 6
VOMITTING – 1,2,4,5
VERTIGO – 3

WEAKNESS, GENERAL – 2,4,7
WEIGHT CONTROL – 1,2,4,7
WEAK LEGS – 7

References

Agrawal, A.L. and Marda, S.P., *Introduction to Acupuncture,* Jaypee Brothers, Delhi.

Bansal, Dr. H.L. and Dr. R.S., *Magneto Therapy Self Help Book,* Jain Publishers.

Bengali, Neville F, Magnet Therapy, *Theory and Practice,* B. Jain Publishers, Delhi.

Bhatia, R., Heal Thyself, *Arnold Associates,* Bombay.

Birla, Ghanshyam Singh and Hamlin, Colette, *Magnet Therapy—The Gentle and Effective Way to Balance Body Systems,* Healing Arts Press, Rochester, Vermont, USA.

Cerney, J.V., *Acupuncture Without Needles,* D.B.Taraporevala and Sons, Bombay.

Chaudhary and Singh, Chumbak Chikitsa, *Acupressure Health Care System,* Jodhpur.

Dewan, A.P., *Healthy Aging,* A.C. Specialist Publishers.

Dewan, A.P., *Food for Health,* Servants of People Society, Delhi.

Denanai, Shudo, *Introduction to Meridian Therapy,* Eastland Press, Seattle, USA.

Gala, Dr D.R., Gala, Dr. Dhiren, Gala, Dr. Sanjay, *Be Your Own Doctor with Magnet Therapy,* Navneet Publications, Mumbai.

Jaggi, Dr. O.P., *Mental Tension and its Cure,* Orient Paperbacks, Vision Books, Delhi.

Luthra, O.P., *Healing without Medicine,* B. Jain Publishers, Delhi.

Modi, Dr. Krishna Murari, *Cure Aches and Pains through Osteopathy,* Osteopathy Clinic, Bombay.

Namikoshi, Toru, *The Complete Book of Shiatsu Therapy,* B.Jain Publishers, Delhi.

Nagendra, Dr. H.R, Nagarathna, Dr. R., *New Perspectives in Stress, Management,* Vivekanand Kendra Yoga Prakashan, Bangalore.

Peeters, Joelle, *An Introduction to Reflexology, Barnes and Noble Books,* Paragon, USA.

Santwani, M.T., *Art of Magnetic Healing,* B. Jain Publishers, Delhi.

Singh, Dr. Attar, *Acupressure – Nature Cure,* Acupressure Health Centre, Chandigarh.

Singh, Dr Sardar Jaswant, *Practical Nature Therapy,* Singh's Nature Cure College and Hospital, Lucknow.

Singh, Dr Rattan, *The Complete Guide to Acupressure,* Acupressure Health Care System, Jodhpur.

Story, Robert T., *Comprehensive Meridian Therapy,* Library of Congress Catalogue Card, USA.

Vora, Devendra, MD, *Health in Your Hands,* Vols I and II, Navneet Publications, Mumbai.

Woo, Park Jae, *A Guide to Sujok Therapy,* Sujok Academy, Jaipur.

Whitaker, Julian MD and Adderly, Brenda, MHA, *The Power of Magnets to Relieve,* Penguin Group, USA.

Yamamoto, Shizuko and McCarty Patrick, *The Acupressure Handbook,* Pustak Mahal, New Delhi.

www.ingramcontent.com/pod-product-compliance
Lightning Source LLC
Chambersburg PA
CBHW051857130726
47987CB00002B/872